Learning From Salmon

LEARNING FROM SALMON

AND OTHER ESSAYS

HERMAN AIHARA

GEORGE OHSAWA MACROBIOTIC FOUNDATION
OROVILLE, CALIFORNIA

Mr. Aihara's works include

Macrobiotics: An Invitation – June 1971
Milk – A Myth of Civilization – November 1971
Seven Macrobiotic Principles – January 1973
Soybean Diet – November 1974
Acid and Alkaline – May 1980
Learning From Salmon – July 1980

George Ohsawa Macrobiotic Foundation
Oroville, California

ISBN 0-918860-37-7

This book is dedicated to Corneliasan, Marie, Jiro and all friends in America, Europe, and Japan.

Acknowledgments

One day in 1979, Sandy Rothman, the editor of GOMF, advised me that we should publish my past writings in a book form. I appreciated the idea but I had no confidence that my writings would be good enough to comprise a book. Nevertheless, I gathered all the old magazines where my writings were printed and gave them to Sandy. To my surprise, he had compiled all my articles already – even some that were not in my memory. A second surprise came when I learned that he and Carl Ferre, the typesetter and book designer for GOMF, had been discussing the publication of this book and had already given it a name. They assured me this will be a good book.

Thus started *Learning From Salmon*, which was created from twenty years of writings. All these have been corrected by my friends and workers of GOMF over the years: Lou Oles, Bill French, Alice Feinberg, Fred Pulver, and Sandy Rothman are a few of them. I have to give my thanks to Carl Ferre for typesetting and design, to Carl Campbell for the cover design, and to Paul Orbuch for the cover photo. The selection of articles and style of writings were chosen and edited by Sandy. Without his enthusiasm, this book would not be realized.

Herman Aihara
February 1980

Preface

In nature, all existence follows a pattern of order. Also in nature's plan there appears from time to time a human being designed to become a natural leader. Often a person must pass through many kinds of life experiences before this capacity becomes obvious; a certain crystallization finally takes place, and from that point there is no question that the ability of clear vision is a permanent possession of the one so designed. Such a one is Herman Aihara.

Herman was born Nobuo Nishiyama in Kyushu, southern Japan, in September of 1920. He was given his American first name by his teacher George Ohsawa, who suggested names for many of his students in order to smooth their acceptance in other countries. Ohsawa was the extraordinary man, synthesizer of philosophies, who introduced the term 'macrobiotic' to the Western world. In Africa, India, Japan, Europe and then the United States he spearheaded the natural foods movement by giving an old Oriental system of health known as *shokuyodo* ('right way of nourishment') the new name of 'macrobiotics' and attracting thousands of followers. When Ohsawa died in 1966, Herman's position as a macrobiotic leader was clarified. With growth and practice his particular skills became refined over the years, and the tumbles of life produced a rare gem.

Along with the many activities of a family man and president of the George Ohsawa Macrobiotic Foundation, Herman Aihara became a compelling writer. In late 1978 and early the next year I re-read many old issues of the *Macrobiotic Monthly* and I realized that some of his best work was in the form of editorials and pieces written for the magazine. In all those issues, the articles by Herman really stood out. They penetrated. But the richness of his insight had reached only a limited number of readers – subscribers to the *Macrobiotic* and their friends. There was a need to put this work into book form. We began to re-work many of the old articles and transscribe some taped material. Herman wrote some new pieces. With the same sense of joy and adventure conveyed in the articles, *Learning From Salmon* took shape.

In this collection of essays, short articles, poems, and lectures it is evident what direction Herman has developed in his teaching. The branches of his flexible mind have taken a special bent in the direction of psychological subjects, and this has been providential for macrobiotics. Techniques for physical health have been well represented in macrobiotic literature, but a shortcoming has been guidance for inner life. This twenty-year span of writing goes a long way toward answering that need. Characteristically, Herman addresses everyday concerns of the mind and spirit with unpretentious practicality and leaves the reader with fresh inspiration. Personal and marital problems, friendship, the struggle to accept and be accepted, the bridging of East and West – these have proven to respond under the warm accuracy of his awareness. Many things are here: pearls of counsel and reflection, philosophical discussion, humorous anecdotes of the macrobiotic movement, personal experiences. Science, religion, politics, health, and nature are explored with a respectful attitude and a creative curiosity.

Herman Aihara has successfully adapted the concept of 'learning from nature' to all facets of life. His is a special gift to observe, learn, and teach the real nature of any subject at hand. It is a great pleasure to present this collection.

Sandy Rothman
April 1980

Contents

Introduction:

Before Learning From Salmon

Macrobiotics was started in Japan about 300 years ago by a scholar, Ekiken Kaibara. He lectured on how to live a long life. Later, his teachings were compiled into a book called *Yojokun* – 'Advice on Longevity.' This most famous advice was: eat less, sleep less, and desire less.

Then about 100 years ago an army doctor named Sagen Ishizuka studied Oriental medicine after learning that his knowledge of Western medicine couldn't cure his kidney disease. He found the sodium/potassium ratio in foods and in our body to create a physical as well as mental balance, and recommended whole brown rice as the best balancing food. Sagen also reached the conclusion, after searching Western medicine for many years, that food is the highest medicine. He realized that all sickness and physical weakness is caused by wrong eating habits. In other words, he established a science of foods for health and happiness. This is called *shokuyo* in Japanese and was later called *macrobiotics* by his student, George Ohsawa. *Shoku* is all matter (or energy – *ki*) which creates and nourishes the perfect man. *Yo* is the deed or way to nourish ourselves, with the knowledge of *shoku*. *Shokuyo* is the right knowledge and deeds which create and nourish the healthy man.

Learning the grain and vegetable diet from Ishizuka, George Ohsawa observed the diet and cured his sickness which had been abandoned by medical doctors. Since then

1

he devoted his life to introducing this diet all over Japan. As he studied more of this diet, he realized the antagonistic complementarity of sodium and potassium in the diet. The plant and animal worlds are nothing but the manifestation of the yin yang principle, which is recognized in the 5000-year-old vast culture of China (the philosophy of Lao Tsu, the *I Ching, Nei Ching,* herbal medicine, moxa, acupuncture). Ohsawa replaced the terms yin and yang for sodium and potassium, using the concepts of modern physics and chemistry instead of the ancient metaphysical concept of yin yang which appeared in the *I Ching* and *Nei Ching.*

When I attended Ohsawa's lecture meetings for the first time around 1940 I was fascinated by his philosophy of yin and yang. I started reading his books and magazines and attended more lectures and seminars. At these seminars Ohsawa served meals consisting of rice, hiziki seaweed, carrot, burdock, and red beans, cooked by his students. I didn't much like those meals and I couldn't eat such meals at my home. I had no interest in brown rice. But I was so much interested in the yin yang philosophy. My classmates laughed at me when I showed my enthusiasm for this philosophy. Some friends even worried about my mentality, because yin and yang was an old and obsolete concept in Japan. My classmates, the future engineers of Sony, Toyota, Datsun, and Toshiba, were so busy digesting 20th century Western science and technology that they had no interest whatever in an old-fashioned Oriental teaching. (Yin and yang was considered by most intellectuals in Japan as an old principle of Chinese superstition called *Eki fortunetelling.*)

In my first year of college I was chosen for the crew of a rowboat race representing my class. I was the heaviest among the crew, so I was positioned as number one – the man who controls the pitch of the rowing. We trained every day for a month at the river running through downtown Tokyo, where the old style of the city remained. It was summertime. It was so hot that I ate shaved ice with syrup (made with sugar, of course) after the training. The races finished and autumn came. When the cool breezes started, I had a tremendous stomach cramp. I couldn't stand up. My parents called a doctor who gave me a drug which stopped the pain immediately. I did the same thing the following year: trained for rowing on the hot days, ate the shaved ice with sugar for a month, and then had stomach cramps again in autumn. A doctor stopped the pain by injecting some painkiller.

At this time I met Ohsawa and read his popular book, *New Dietetic Medicine* (Japanese version of *Zen Macrobiotics*). I realized the cause of my stomach cramp was eating too much shaved ice and sugar syrup. Both are very yin; ice is yin because it is cold, sugar because it is the opposite of salt. Sugar stops the appetite or inhibits the action of the stomach. In my case, ice and sugar weakened my stomach. When the yin season began, the cool breezes stimulated the stomach muscles to secrete the yang hormone called acetylcholine. When muscles are weak (yin) and expanded (yin), as with the condition I had, contraction is difficult. In other words, yin muscles resist natural contraction, and stress and strain builds up. Finally, the contracting effect of the hormone overwhelms, and the muscle contracts. However, it does so in a very clumsy way. It cramps. This is a yin contraction, while the normal contraction is yang. Thinking that since the cause of the cramp was yin and salt is yang, I started taking salt for my stomach. Soon it was better. Then I thought I knew macrobiotics. I thought I knew the secret of macrobiotics – that is to say, the use of salt. What a silly mentality.

After these experiences came my graduation year. I spent many hours of my school days at the laboratory, experimenting for the graduation thesis. I often cooked meals by myself at the laboratory with much wild grasses, oil, and salt, thinking that was the macrobiotic cooking. Such a diet damaged my stomach and intestines, stopping the assimilation of nutrition. I became thinner and thinner. My parents started to worry. Friends advised me to stop my diet or belief; I didn't listen because I thought I was doing the right thing – the macrobiotic diet. I was active in school sports even though I had lost much weight. Then came the draft examination. I failed. I was too weak and too skinny. My friends were surprised, since I was one of the most athletic students, playing many school sports. However, I still didn't realize I was sick.

After graduate school I worked in my father's factory. My parents were so worried about my skinny condition that they sent me to my mother's native community, to a friend's country home, believing I was tubercular. When all young people were either fighting at the front or working in factories, I was travelling from one place to another without specific aim or responsibility. Having graduated from the engineering school of a reputable university, I should have been working in a very important industrial position for Japan, who was fighting with the world Allies. The onetime bright student was like a disabled, retarded man in such a most important time for the nation. My parents were very disappointed, and blamed macrobiotics as the cause of my sickness. Only I knew the real cause of my sickness. It was arrogance. I was arrogant! I thought I understood macrobiotics but my practice was unwise. Under my family circumstances, to recover from sickness it was best to give up my intention to be macrobiotic. It took about three years to completely recover after I gave up macrobiotics. (Now, I could probably cure such a condition in three months with the macrobiotic diet.) From this experience I learned that an unwise or fanatic application of macrobiotics could be dangerous. The study of life is a lifelong work. Since then I never thought I have learned macrobiotics enough. That experience made me humble. I try to always listen to others' opinions and then humbly establish my opinion.

When the war ended in 1945, I had recovered from a sickness of the stomach and intestines – probably ulcers. I worked in my father's factory. I was a college graduate, but I had failed in macrobiotics. I was eating at home, anything my mother served for me. She cooked fish twice a day, white rice, and used sugar in cooking. Foods were very scarce at that time but we could get anything we wanted through the black market.

I became extremely yang in behavior. I started to learn American social dancing at the newly opened dance halls. Social dance was a new fashion after American forces occupied Japan. When people were starving to death just after the war, I was a playboy, chasing sexy girls at various dance halls.

My father worried about my behavior and hurried my marriage. I married because my parents were agreed, but I myself was not much attracted to her. My wife committed suicide before our marriage passed one year. It was the end of autumn. She climbed a mountain alone, drank poison, and died without giving anyone her reasons. No one but I understood how she could do such a thing. The reason was her difficulty in coping with my adoptive mother and complicated family structure (we were living with my very yang stepmother and my brother-in-law and his only daughter). Since my mother controlled domestic matters and she relied on my brother-in-law rather than me because he was my boss and a good businessman, my wife was never relaxed in our home. She couldn't see independence in my future. Hers was very much a Japanese expression of love. She warned and advised me by giving up her life.

I was shocked and depressed for a long time. I lost my mind for a month. How pitiful a man I was. My wife could not rely on me. I should have been the sort of man who could carry the burden of a wife and family, at the very least. I didn't know what to do.

At that point I decided to make myself an independent man and I chose Mr. George Ohsawa as my life's teacher. I

went to his macrobiotic school and asked him to let me stay.
He said I could stay in his school. It was unique, not only in
his teaching but also as far as the school administration was
concerned. There was neither requirement for admission nor
tuition. Anybody could stay and study. Students had to eat
meals served twice daily, cooked by a girl who is now one
of the best macrobiotic cooking teachers in Japan. This was
not exactly a requirement; there was no need for such a requirement, because one who didn't eat meals there would
not want to stay there anyway.

In fact, there was one sort of requirement. Students had to
answer Mr. Ohsawa's questions by themselves, not by way
of a textbook or dictionary. The curriculum was in two parts –
one was a mental education (yin) and the other was physical
(yang). The school day began with sweeping, washing, and
putting things in order. This was not merely an exercise in
yangization but it taught us orderliness. Ohsawa emphasized
this work because orderliness is one of the most important
conditions for health. Next came a lecture by Mr. Ohsawa –
the main part of the curriculum. The subjects covered all
fields: foreign and domestic news, science, medicine, economics, politics, modern living, business, industry, astronomy,
cosmology, religion, sociology, and more. In the afternoons,
students worked in the school or outside of it. Even this came
within the scope of his teaching since they had to submit
a report and get his criticism or remark. This was followed
at night by solitary study or discussion in a group. Sleeping
was another part of the curriculum: a short, fast, deep sleep
was a sign of the good health which students wanted to acquire.

All the lectures were given to exercise our ability to think –
the path to higher judgment. It did not matter which subject
Mr. Ohsawa chose – from physics to metaphysics, from matter to non-matter, from the biography of Gandhi to that of
Benjamin Franklin. His lesson was always the understanding

of the order of the universe, justice, freedom, and eternal love. During my one month stay, he never taught us symptomatic Western medicine, Oriental medicine, or treatments for sickness such as ginger compresses, albi plasters, etc. Physical diagnoses were left completely to our self-study. His only teaching was for us to understand and acquire infinite freedom, absolute justice, and eternal love.

Finally, the student himself decided whether or not he was graduated from Ohsawa's teaching. Most students bypassed graduation and just left the school. However, they were welcomed to return at any time. What made a graduate? He who understood the principles of macrobiotics and a-chieved health and happiness in his life was the graduate. Freedom from all constraints or troubles such as sickness, poverty, hate, fear, etc., was the certificate of graduation. That was why graduation was not controlled as in the usual school. The students who graduated easily often met trouble or became unhappy, and realized they needed more study.

During my stay at Ohsawa's school, I was so depressed that my mind was out in space. I didn't do anything or help in the tasks such as cleaning rooms, cooking meals, shipping books and magazines, or writing and editing for Ohsawa's monthly magazine. I just ate, slept, and listened very seriously to Ohsawa's lectures. Although I was his laziest student, Ohsawa blamed nothing for my laziness because he knew I was serious about learning what he tried to teach. I was very serious. I was looking for how to live, and I found it in one month's time. I made a big discovery. I found myself. Christ said, "If you know yourselves you will be known, and you will know that you are the sons of the Living Father. But if you do not know yourselves then you are in poverty and you are poverty." (The Gospel according to Thomas.) What I found in a month's time is who I am. I didn't learn meridians or compresses – I can't teach those techniques. I can teach one thing: who you are. To learn 'who I am' you don't need any books. All of a sudden, you are there.

At the same time I learned two more things: "Everyone is happy; if not, it is his own fault" (Epictetus) and that the food you eat is one of the most important factors for your health and happiness.

I returned home to the job in my father's factory. My character and behavior looked the same, but my understanding of life had completely changed. I became more and more an adventurer, and my desire to be independent became stronger. Finally, I decided to leave Japan forever to see other worlds and build my independence. Decision makes action. I abandoned my fortune and my parents and made the fees for the transportation from Japan to the United States by second class in a cargo boat, $360 even at that time. I landed in San Francisco with great joy and curiosity in 1952 at the age of 32. My new life had started.

Since then I have experienced many difficulties and much sadness: immigration troubles, causing me to leave this country three times, twice to the Bahamas and once to Europe; the death of my parents (they gave me lots of love but I gave them only worry); the death of my babies, caused by my ignorance and arrogance; and finally my second wife's sickness. I not only overcame all these difficulties but established a happy and wonderful life. This is due to my first tragedy and to the teaching of George Ohsawa.

In 1960 I started publishing the first *Macrobiotic News*, which consisted mostly of Ohsawa's articles and lecture notes. After his death, Lou Oles continued the magazine and books with me; after Lou's death, I continued the publications. This book is a compilation of my shorter writings over the last twenty years.

It is my sincere hope that my learning from George Ohsawa can be of some help to you and that you might enjoy the whole of your life instead of living in fear, resentment, desperation, and anger.

Herman Aihara
February, 1980

Learning
From Salmon

November 1964

Thanksgiving 1964

Cold and hunger are the forces that produce
    warmth and fullness.
From poverty we can become rich.
      Sickness spurs our search for health.
Health or wealth by birth is not ours –
    it is our parents' gift to us.
As such, it will disappear sooner or later.

You must be the creator of your own
    health or wealth.
If you understand this fully, you will have
    no enemies and will be without hatred.
Since enemies challenge you,
    they build your strength.
For this, they deserve only thanks
    and gratitude.
This is the true life of man.

Is there any such human on Earth today?
    Yes — you.
You give thanks for everything today.
    You have no hatred, no enemy.
    You are all-embracing.
At this moment, you are wholeness.

Give thanks for your weakness, sickness,
  poverty, exclusiveness, and arrogance.
Through them you have the biggest chance
  to be healthy, strong, rich,
  all-embracing and humble.

America Was Defeated

The peace agreement between America and Vietnam was finally signed on January 28th, 1973. America bowed to Vietnam after all, losing 5,000 young Americans, injuring 300,000 soldiers, spending $150 billion on arms and explosives, including chemical poisons, and dropping 7 million tons of bombs, which is three times the total bombs dropped in World War II.

Why did America – the strongest nation in the world – have to bow to Vietnam, which was armed with little more than a pistol? There are no wars in man's history which reveal the difference in armed strength so drastically. Vietnam was a mouse in front of a cat or a rabbit before a lion.

Why was America defeated by such a weak nation?

The reason is clear to me. America had no justice in fighting Vietnam, and American youths felt the injustice in the Vietnam War. American youth had no fighting spirit at the front or at home. They protested against the draft, made riots, and escaped into drugs because they saw injustice.

Contrary to the Americans, the Vietnamese had a reason to fight. They have had enough exploitations by foreigners – China, France, and Japan – in their history. Those exploitations made them make up their minds to fight for their freedom and independence.

Also contrary to the Americans, the Vietnamese had the endurance to withstand long fighting. They lived on the poorest foods which many American nutritionists consider nutritionally insufficient.

The defeat of America by Vietnam is the greatest miracle in the 20th century. The cause of this must be thoroughly investigated, and man should learn from it. Otherwise America's name will remain as a mere murderer in man's history. If we learn a great lesson from this defeat, the defeated will be the winner.

Happy New Year 1974

In Japan, the New Year's Day is a most joyous day for children as well as adults. It is not only joyous but also highly spiritual. Every house and town is filled with spiritual serenity. Every house entrance is decorated with rice straw (*shimenawa*) which probably suggests that each house would be enshrined with gods. In the morning, the streets are completely quiet until noon, because every home is celebrating the New Year Dinner.

The head of the household sits in the main room with formal kimono, and other members of the family salute him with congratulations of the New Year, and receive *toso sake* which probably started originally as a medicinal drink for long life.

Foods for the New Year Day (or week) are completely macrobiotic, except in modern use where monosodium glutamate and sugar are used. There is always mochi soup, including various vegetables depending on local customs. Town people use fish cakes and nori with bonita soup stock. I remember that I used to eat lots of mochi, more than ten pieces in our meal; albi; mashed sweet potato; black beans; burdock; lotus root; kombu; azuki beans; carrot; small fish; etc., all of which are cooked before New Year's Day and served at each meal from storage boxes. Therefore, the women minimize their cooking for at least three days of the New Year.

After brunch, the children go out to play or play indoors.

The adults become busy entertaining visitiors who come for the New Year celebration. This celebration continues for at least three days (or it did when I was a child). We felt very much that the New Year was here and now. But today, in America, there is neither any special feeling nor any distinction of changes. A New Year passes by as another day of life. There is no excitement. There is no plan for the New Year.

However, a New Year's Day is only meaningful when one recalls the past year and sets a plan for the coming year. Our life is balancing yin and yang – passive and active. At the close of the year we figure out whether we have been eating or doing too much to the yin side or the yang side. Then, on New Year's Day, we may plan a balancing schedule according to our past yin yang intake or activity. Otherwise a yin person may continue to become more yin and a yang person may continue further yang until sicknesses, accidents, or misfortunes happen.

In the old Japanese calendar, a New Year's Day is the first day of spring (at the beginning of February). Counting 88 days from this New Year, farmers soaked rice seeds in water for planting. Therefore, the New Year's Day was really important as a planning day for the year. If farmers plant rice too early, it may die from the frost. If they plant too late, there will not be enough hot weather for it to grow.

In the modern world, our life is detached from the soil and so from seasonal change. In order to go back to natural living, we should start to think of the importance of New Year's Day. And we should plan our schedule of the coming year so that we will be able to harvest in the autumn.

An Introduction to Spiritual Japan

The Japanese mentality or spiritual world of Japan is strange, confusing, and mystical to almost all foreigners. Japanese people who live in Japan are not aware of this because they cannot see themselves from the outside. However, I, a Japanese living in America for more than twenty years, think the Japanese mentality is strange if not confusing. Therefore, I understand that it is quite natural when the foreigner who visits Japan misunderstands the mentality and culture.

Lafcadio Hearn, who loved Japan so much that he married a Japanese woman and became a Japanese citizen, wrote in his *Japan, An Attempt At Interpretation:* "Long ago, the best and dearest Japanese friend I ever had said to me, a little before his death: 'When you find, in four or five years more, that you cannot understand the Japanese at all, then you will begin to know something about them.' "

Similar thought was expressed by George Ohsawa, the founder of the American macrobiotic movement. He wrote in a small article entitled *The Mentality of a Nation is Imperceptible:* "Mentality is invisible, as are character and personality. Mentality, character, personality, and even mood or emotion are nothing but an expression of judgment (wisdom) in a relative, physical, and finite world, and that expression varies according to circumstances. If we want to determine a nation's character, we must study and understand the na-

16

tion's philosophy, its conception of the world, and its logic – upon which all judgment depends. It is extremely difficult, if not impossible, for Occidentals to understand the character of any Oriental peoples. Why? Because the philosophy or world concept and logic of the East are completely opposite to that of the West."

He continues, "I have read many books treating of Japan – of Japanese people and their culture, their art, all of them written by more or less outstanding Occidental authors. Each time I read such a book I am profoundly shocked. I am a complete stranger to the Japanese subject they write about, whether people, civilization, culture, or philosophy. Then I say to myself, 'I must explain . . .' That is why I am still writing, still trying to explain our mentality, as I promised Professor Levi-Bruhl thirty years ago."

To outward appearances, Japan is the most Westernized country in the East. Japanese people wear Western style clothing, shirts, and shoes. Their living standards are higher than some of the Westerners. Their industry and technology have surpassed that of the Western countries who taught Japan about technology. They not only have adopted the Western style of materialistic civilization, but also mastered Western religions, at least on the surface. There are all kinds of religion in Japan now. For example, there are about 4,000 Christian churches with members totalling about 700,000 with denominations including Catholic, Protestant, Seventh Day Adventist, The Salvation Army, etc. There are also followers of Baha'i, Mohammed, Hinduism, Tibetan Buddhism, and others.

Furthermore, there are more than thirty modern religions, some of them having more than fifteen million followers (such as Soka Gakakai). However, their strongest faith is tied to Shintoism and Buddhism. In other words, the Japanese still maintain their old mentality and have not modernized yet. According to recent statistics, Shinto had seventy million followers, while Buddhism had seventy-five million believers. These statistics show the strange fact that the sum of the believers of Shintoism and Buddhism surpasses the total population of Japan. This fact can be easily explained. They believe in Shintoism and Buddhism at the same time. They offer foods to their ancestors in Shinto style, yet give Buddhist chants to their ancestors. Rice, salt, water, and vegetables are a common offering at the Shinto shrines while fruits and cakes are the offering at the Buddhist altar of the ancestors. A Christian may marry in front of a Shinto shrine, and a Shintoist may receive a Buddhist funeral. It is commonly accepted that a Buddhist ceremony is for the dead and the Shinto ceremony is for the living.

For some foreigners, this attitude may cause bewilderment. In fact, an understanding of this attitude is one of the key points in understanding the Japanese mentality and their spiritual world. Japan is a rare country in which there has been no religious discrimination. There have been no wars between religions in Japan such as between Jews and Arabs, Mohammedans and Hindus, Catholics and Protestants. The reason for this nondiscrimination is based on their belief that all religions are one and all spiritual worlds are one. This belief is called the Japanese Religion (Nihonism) by Isaiah Ben-Dasan, author of *The Japanese and the Jews*.

Another important characteristic of the spiritual concept or faith of the Japanese is the ancestor worship Lafcadio Hearn mentioned in his *Japan, An Attempt At Interpretation*. Ancestor worship in Japan consists of about three principles in its basic belief.

1. The dead remain in this world – haunting their tombs, and also their former homes, and sharing invisibly in the life of their descendents.

2. All the dead become gods, in the sense of acquiring supernatural power; but they retain the character which distinguished them during life.

3. The happiness of the dead depends upon the respectful service rendered them by the living, and the happiness of the living depends upon the fulfillment of pious duty to the dead.

These are a scientific and analytical civilized person's views on primitive Japanese mentality. However, most Japanese do not see themselves in this way because the world of the dead is not entirely a separate world from the living. The world of the dead is a continuation of the living. Therefore, there is no death in the sense the English word means. When one's physical body disappears in the invisible world, then one is called dead but to the traditional Japanese he is not dead. He is living in the invisible world which is called anti-matter in modern physics. Therefore, the living people talk to the dead and offer food.

In reality, the Japanese conceive that the world where the dead are living is the real world and the world where we see and sense is the false world because it is ephemeral and limited. To the Japanese, the offering of food is not a duty but it is a pleasure and joy – just like giving food to the family is mother's joy. Here again we realize the basic concept or mentality of the Japanese. That is to say, life and death are one. Without understanding this concept, one cannot understand the *harakiri* or *kamikaze* of Japanese soldiers or samurais. The ultimate aim of the swordsmanship of Japanese fencing is to reach the realization of the concept of oneness of life and death.

The third basic concept or mentality of the Japanese is the monistic view of God and man which differs from the concepts of Christianity and Judaism. I believe all religion as well as primitive faith originally had this basic concept that God and man are one. For the Japanese, who fortunately have been living with an abundant supply of sunlight, water, fertile land and green woods, nature was lovely and life was joyous and happy – until Buddhism brought them a negativistic view of life: life is suffering.

Since then, the Japanese view of life has changed to a more negativistic and pessimistic one. However, Buddhism enriched Japanese mentality by giving a view of the ephemerality of life or the philosophical concept that everything changes.

Consequently, Japanese mentality was influenced greatly by two views – joy and sorrow, optimism and pessimism, yin and yang. One of these views appears dominant in certain periods of time, location, and individual personality. However, their overall mentality, behavior, ethics, or religion can be summarized into one – appreciation of the creator of life and nature, which is rather a Shintoistic view. This creator was considered as God when people lived closely with nature.

God is the loving mother and father instead of a scolding or punishing 'almighty.' However, the development of living standards separated man from nature, which is God. We began living less in connection with nature and more with man-made conveniences and commercialism, forgetting the importance of right foods. Man's ego and conceptual thinking grew. As a result, man cannot see oneness. We separated God from Man.

Today it is difficult to find the people or the land which Lafcadio Hearn so much admired. He wrote, "I fancy that if we were able to enter for a moment into the vanished life of some old Greek city, we should find the domestic religion there not less cheerful than the Japanese home-cult remains today. I imagine the Greek children, three thousand years ago, must have watched, like the Japanese children of today, for a chance to steal some of the good things offered to the ghosts of the ancestors and I fancy that Greek parents must have chided their children quite as gently as Japanese parents in this era of Meiji, mingling reproof with instruction, and hinting of weird possibility."

However, any good and unprejudiced observer will be able to see this heartwarming ancestor worship and life which is based on a monistic view of man and God, religions, life and death, etc. This finding will open you to another dimension of life as mentioned by Arnold Toynbee, an English historian, who in his last visit to Japan about ten years ago said Japan was his second motherland where he finds mental ease and peace.

March 1961, New York City

The President's Greeting

It is a wonderful feeling – and I am deeply grateful – to be welcomed by all of you upon our return from Europe. . . . And, more, to be welcomed by the news that you have elected me president of the Ohsawa Foundation.

I am touched by this evidence of your confidence in me, but fear that I may not be able to discharge this great duty with the intelligence and good judgment such a job demands. I worry for fear I may do something that might retard or hinder the development of the Ohsawa movement, a movement which is most revolutionary, one of the most revolutionary in our history in every field – science, economy, education, religion, medicine, and politics. I think the president of this Foundation should be a distinguished man, and I am not such a man. The only way I see for us to proceed is to work together, each of us working with the other, and do the best we are capable of doing; to cooperate in this enormous job and do our best to further the purposes of the Ohsawa Foundation. I am an insignificant man; with your help and constant cooperation, perhaps we can forge ahead.

For this reason, may I ask all of you for your suggestions and criticism as to the way and manner in which the affairs of the Foundation are being conducted. Please speak out, freely and openly; let us know if we are doing something wrong, and tell us how to do it right. Give the Foundation and all its members the benefits of your judgment. It may be better than ours. In any case, we need your help. Please get in touch with any or all of us with your suggestions and criticisms. We shall appreciate anything you have to offer.

In September 1952, one Japanese boy landed at San Francisco. He was alone, had no acquaintances or friends, and could understand and speak but a few words of English. However, strangely enough, he seemed very happy in such a state, and was not worried about the future. This sense of happiness and freedom from worry was due entirely to his diet, and a spiralic conception of the universe.

Eight years passed, and this same boy was aboard the Holland American liner leaving New York harbor for Europe in September 1960. He was on his way to Europe, accompanied by his wife and two children this time. Many friends bid him goodbye at the dock; but, too, there were many friends to greet him in Europe. What changes had there been in the life of this boy who landed in San Francisco only a few short years ago? Some of the changes were unhappy ones: the death of his parents far away, the sickness of his wife, and the death of their two babies. Nevertheless, the young man was happy to recall the events of the past eight years. The memory was inspiring.

Memory? What is memory? Memory that has no time, no space; memory that can be recalled any time, any place; old and new at the same time; memories from Japan, America, and Europe. What a wonderful mechanism the memory is. We live in the ocean of memory – memory that exists everywhere and at any time; omniscient, omnipresent. "God made man in his own image," we read, and image is memory. A man grows trillions of times in his mother's womb by this image; that is to say, man has his memory, his plan of growth. But then everything has memory – even the plants, the stones, the water, all animals, everything from atoms to planets. But memory through education or experience is not memory. It is an illusion, since that kind of memory depends upon perception or senses, which is different in each person according to his capacity, training, intelligence, etc. That is not true memory. As long as we have our being in memory we are happy, healthy, and free. To recall this memory is to be happy. To act through this memory is freedom. To live in this memory is health.

What did I get in Europe? In five months I met many macrobiotic friends, saw beautiful macrobiotic restaurants and clinics in Belgium, France, Italy, Germany, Switzerland, and England. The Lima macrobiotic factory produces three tons of macaroni and spaghetti a day; sanarant *Ceres* is filled with so-called incurable patients; and the restaurants *Au Riz Dore* and *Longue Vie* are both making people healthier and happier by the day. Seeing all this favorable progress in Europe confirmed my belief in the destiny of the macrobiotic movement in America. Still, this was not what I got from my trip to Europe.

After his study in China, Dogen, the foremost Japanese Zen priest, said: "What I learned in China is that the eye is horizontal and the nose is vertical." That is, in substance, what I got from my five months in Europe.

Americans and Europeans write their name and address from the individual to the nation. The Japanese write theirs from the nation to the individual:

Western Style	Japanese Style
Herman Aihara	Japan
44 West 96th St.	Tokyo, Katushika
New York, NY	Tateishi
U.S.A.	341
Earth (we'll need this in the future)	Herman Aihara

How come this big difference? The difference comes because of the difference in the way of thinking.

Western thinking starts from the individual, part, or section and goes towards infinity. That is why Occidental science meets confusion in the end, aiming truth in the eternal future. Oriental thinking, on the contrary, starts from infinity, oneness, and truth and proceeds towards the individual, part, or section; that is to say, via deduction. Oriental thinking knows the answer, then confirms it in actual cases.

Each method has advantages and disadvantages. If both ways of thinking were combined and understood, a new science and a new civilization would begin. Only such a combination can solve our human crisis.

That is what I got from my trip to Europe.

Macrobiotic Beginnings in the United States

At the first American macrobiotic lectures held in Long Island in 1960, one psychiatric doctor asked George Ohsawa if he would come back to New York for a summer camp. Ohsawa said, "If your attraction is strong enough, I will." So this Dr. Kronemeyer organized the first summer camp, at Long Island, New York. Ohsawa then flew back from Paris and we had the first camp. It lasted two months. Every day, every day many interesting people came.

One of them was Red Buttons. His wife had leukemia, and they heard somewhere about Ohsawa – a strange, Oriental doctor, teaching Oriental philosophy and diet. They came to camp: "Please cure my leukemia." So, Ohsawa took care of Red Buttons' wife, recommending pheasant meat – the most yang meat. Red Buttons was such an interesting man – so funny. One day he spoke in front of us. Everybody laughed and laughed and laughed. He sang a song for us one night, a Jewish song, at a campfire gathering like this. He sang a Jewish song and, surprisingly, his Jewish song is a Japanese song! Exactly the same as a Japanese song.

At that time I was managing our store in New York City, selling Japanese gift items and macrobiotic food. The first macrobiotic food store in the States. Dr. W., a learned medical doctor, came to our meeting, studied macrobiotic techniques, and started teaching his patients. His patients came to my store every day, buying food. Ten people came every day. It was growing so fast. If even one doctor recommends macrobiotics, this country would change very easily. At that time one doctor recommended it. However, after teaching macrobiotics, patients didn't come back to him! So he stopped. He was also afraid the AMA would kick him out of the organization. His wife was an alcoholic; as soon as he started macrobiotics, his wife stopped her alcoholism. They were very happy. Then, when he stopped macrobiotics, his wife went back to alcohol. They divorced. Very sad.

At this same time, in 1960, I had difficulties with the famous American Immigration Office. I was deported many times. For five or six years I had been fighting with immigration officers; they said: "You should leave this country immediately, this is the final notice," etc. So as soon as summer camp was over I went to Europe, with my wife and two kids, to change my visa. I went on *The Amsterdam* to Holland, Belgium, France, and Italy. First I stayed in Belgium one month. There I bought a car; I didn't know much about automobiles at that time, so I bought an English Ford. Belgium does not manufacture its own cars, so I bought this English Ford secondhand, an old car. As soon as I had the car I started driving toward France and Italy. Passing by Paris, I heard a sound from the front wheel: the bearing was broken. So I stopped at a garage and asked them to fix it. They said they had no parts, that I would have to wait three days. The part came, it was fixed, and I drove away. Then the muffler broke. I asked many places, but always: "There is no part, cannot fix." Arriving in Italy, climbing up the Alps, the car would not go up. So I went to the bottom and stayed overnight; the nest morning I put the gear speed higher and made it to the top of the hill. This way we crossed the Alps and went to Italy. When we arrived at Rome, they said the engine was no good. So I had to stay at the mechanic's while he fixed the engine. The parts had to come from England – we stayed three weeks. During that time I taught macrobiotic cooking to the people in Rome.

Upon my arrival in Belgium from New York I had applied
for a visa to go back to America but they hesitated. Then, I
went out travelling. Five months later I returned to Belgium
and asked again if my visa had arrived from the U.S. They
said no. I thought, they are checking my background and I
have been underground in the U.S. four or five years; this is
not good. So I decided to try Antwerp, another port where
there was an American consulate, instead of Brussels. I applied for a transit visa – that means passing by the U.S., only
staying a day or so en route to Japan. I was immediately
given a transit visa to the States. I could return to America.
Since then I have stayed nineteen years. This you can do.
After all, each of us is a visitor to the planet Earth with a
transit visa from the Infinite World. I left England on the
Queen Mary. This ship is now in Long Beach. It was very
bad. Traveling third class, the room is at the bottom of the
ship – very bad air, no circulation. And the food: it is such
a big ship, food is preserved for many months. Rice was
rotten. That's the kind of food you have to eat on the Queen
Mary. I returned on the last voyage of the Queen Mary. I'm
happy it is now a museum.

When I arrived in New York, I heard I had been elected
president of the macrobiotic organization. I was elected without knowing it. I started publishing a magazine – I think I
called it the *Macrobiotic News*. It was mostly Ohsawa's lectures, offset printed. Since then I have been doing the same
thing. In 1961, after I returned to New York, Ohsawa came
again and lectured, and in the summertime we had the second
summer camp. This time we were at Watsboro, in the Catskill
Mountains, outside of New York.

Ohsawa was very sick – why I don't know; he was very sick,
but he lectured anyway. Before his lecture time he was bent
over, but nobody realized he was sick. After the lecture he
went back to bed. One time he asked me, "Please get whiskey."
I told him, today's Sunday, no stores are open. He said,

"Please get." He asked me to get yogurt. He was experimenting! When sick, he always experimented. He is a man enjoying sickness. I never met a man who encouraged his sickness. After 40 years of macrobiotics, I'm sure he knew how to cure it. But he didn't try to cure. At the next lecture he said, "Mmm. Yogurt very yin." That was Ohsawa. A very amazing man.

After the 1961 camp, the world situation was very tense. Kruschchev was the premier of Russia and Kennedy was president of the United States. Kruschchev was planning to build nuclear weapons in Cuba, transporting Russian-made nuclear materials to Cuba. Kennedy declared he would fight if Russia proceeded with the delivery. Hearing this news Ohsawa told us, "Atomic war is very close. We have to prepare for war. You should evacuate New York – it will be Russia's first target." So, all macrobiotic students gathered in downtown New York – two or three thousand people arrived and gathered in a big hall to discuss what to do. One said, we should go to Australia. One said west, another said south, another north. We all discussed. One, an atomic engineer, checked a report from the Atomic Energy Commission which said there was no safe place in the United States in case of nuclear attack. Winds would carry the fallout. However, according to this report, the least fallout would be in the Sacramento Valley of California. In all of the U.S., it is the only large valley surrounded by mountains on all sides. So, any wind dropping fallout would stay outside of the Sacramento Valley (unless the bomb was dropped inside the Sacramento Valley! . . . *laughter* . . .). So finally we decided to move to the Sacramento Valley. We checked to see what town we would move to. We discussed every day, every night. Three members were elected to fly to San Francisco to check the towns: Al Bauman, Bill Salant, and myself. Bill was a presidential economic advisor – a high official of government – and Al had been a music professor at Columbia University. He was teaching many people a very interesting music therapy and introduced many people to the macrobiotic diet. Later, after moving to California, Al became president of Synanon.

The three of us flew from New York to San Francisco, hired a car, and drove up to the Sacramento Valley towards Mt. Shasta. We drove up and down and checked all the towns. We decided Chico would be a suitable town; it was small but large enough, with a university, radio and television stations, and cultural activities. We flew back to New York with our report. We told all the macrobiotic members we decided to move to Chico – how many will go together? Fifteen families decided to go – 36 people, including babies. Everybody packed, got tents and sleeping bags, packed cars, and gathered outside New York City. We started traveling. As soon as they heard the news, all the New York newspapers wrote on the front page: "Modern 20th Century Exodus." One reporter always followed us – our movement was always reported. Very funny.

We usually drove 300 miles a day. We would arrive at a campground, put up tents, cook together, eat together, and not sleep together! (*Laughter.*) Then at night we would have meetings to plan the next day, where to stop and camp out next. Early the next morning we packed up the cars and drove another 300 miles. Every day, every day. We never stopped at motels – always camping grounds. It took about 16 days to reach California. One day around Nebraska or Missouri, in the famous Midwest, we had a big storm. We were at a lakeside. Most everybody went to a motel and only a few families stayed at the campground. The next day, it was the most beautiful morning we ever had.

We continued on to California and arrived at Lake Tahoe. We had left New York around September 1, and arrived in the middle of September at Lake Tahoe. We stayed a few days at Lake Tahoe – Emerald Bay. A television reporter came to our campground and interviewed us. Always! (*Laughter.*)

Then, we arrived in Chico. This trip was very, very fascinating. We had no accidents. No injuries. No sickness. Nobody complained. We had the happiest trip we ever had. On the way we had discussed what to do in Chico, a place we had never been. What kind of jobs would we have? We decided to start a macrobiotic foods production factory and distribution company. We founded a company and named it Chico San. Chico is the name of the town, *san* is Japanese word for intimacy: Chico San. Nobody knew, *Chiiko* is my wife's name.

To form Chico San we gathered investments from 15 people – one gave $10,000, one gave $500, and so on. This was the beginning of the first macrobiotic production company and distributor in the U.S. The first store was the basement of a small shop. I imported the first merchandise from Japan: miso, tamari, wakame, hiziki, dried fish, etc., and we opened the store. When the first merchandise arrived we had an open house and invited the townspeople. The Chico townspeople came to the first macrobiotic store: "What is this? What is this? What is this?" Everyone was curious. They had never seen these things before. One man looked at small fish. "You eat this fish? You eat *eye?!*"

I was the baker. Why I became a baker I don't know – I never ate bread. Oh, a little bit, but almost none; in Japan there was no bread at that time. I became a bread baker. I baked Ohsawa bread. (You know Ohsawa bread? Only old macrobiotic knows.) Whole wheat flour and cooked brown rice, mixed into a dough with no yeast. Three inches long, one inch thick: one pound! Heavy – like a golden nugget! That bread, two or three days later you cannot cut. You need a hammer. So, we decided to take orders – order-made bread! You never heard of order-made bread; at Chico San we had order-made bread. One place ordered 2, another 6, another 6. Somebody ordered 12. The truck driver liked it – he chewed while driving. I also made whole wheat bread with a little yeast, no sugar or preservative; much fiber. After baking we took the bread to the Bay Area: San Francisco, San Rafael, Oakland. We took it to health food stores and asked them to buy. They said they would sell on consignment. I came back one week later – all the bread was returned. That was 1961 and 1962. That's the start of macrobiotics in this country.

After we left New York, the remaining people organized and kept the Ohsawa Foundation. They had a store. An unfortunate accident happened – one customer got very sick and died. The FDA came in and closed the store. In Chico, they came to inspect our store. Every item was checked, every label. They took one book and one package back. The book was *Zen Macrobiotics*. What was the package? Not fish, salt, miso, mu tea, rice, bread, rice cakes, bancha tea, or umeboshi. It was the toothpowder, dentie. Dentie! That is a medical name – we cannot use the name, dentie! So, we don't use dentie any more. Since then, we had to separate the Foundation and the food business. In this country, the FDA law requires that if you teach a certain diet, you cannot sell the products. Until then, Chico San and the Foundation were one: everyone worked at both. So we separated Chico San and the Foundation. Lou Oles was elected the first president of the Ohsawa Foundation, and Bob Kennedy became president of Chico San. I was working at Chico San. Nobody knew macrobiotic food in this country; to sell food, we always had to give cooking classes. We taught in San Francisco, Los Angeles, Palm Springs, San Diego. That way we developed more customers, little by little. We sold very little food. Most of the customers were our own 15 families – 36 people mostly buying our food. So, there was very little business, and we had no salary. For 3 years we had no salary.

Bob Kennedy, Dick Smith, and Irv Hirsch were musicians. Friday and Saturday were their special days – they went to bars and played trumpet. They had an income. Each time they played . . . twenty or thirty dollars. But I had no income. So, sometimes I went to the orchards and picked peaches or prunes, famous California prunes. I picked California peaches and Sunkist California oranges. One day I went to pick prunes. When the prunes are a little bit greenish, before ripe, they shake the tree. All the prunes drop on the ground, and you pick them up and put them in the bin. The bin size is 3′ by 3′ by 3′. They paid $7.50 for a full one. It took me a whole day to pick up enough prunes to fill one bin. I cried. Hot sunshine. Scorching heat. $7.50. I saw many Mexican children also picking: $7.50 a bin. I made the same. They are faster. One family came, earning thirty or forty dollars. I cried.

One day I went to pick peaches. It was very hot. Starting at 5:00 in the morning, that was very good – cool. An orchard at 5:00 in the morning is very cold. As soon as the sun came up it became hot, hot, hot. In front of me, big Freestone peaches, hanging. I eat one. I eat another one. I eat another one. I eat another one. I thought peaches are very yin. Now I know peaches are yin. I don't much like peaches – no more. I ate enough.

So, business was very bad. I had seen rice cakes in Belgium and had helped to make them on a very primitive machine. I advised, why don't we make rice cakes here, maybe we can sell more. So we imported a rice cake machine from Japan. Very simple: you sit, put in the rice, press down, release. Then take out one rice cake, put in more rice, press down – another one. Then we got another rice cake machine, then two more. We had four machines. Bob Kennedy was very ingenious. He added a bar connecting all four machines so that one lever operated all four at one time. Press down, release; four rice cakes at one time. Orders started coming in. We had three shifts making rice cakes.

But the four rice cake machines produced a strong power – you would be surprised at so much power. I am small, and each time pressing down I had to jump up. Then it releases with so much power. I hurt my shoulder. So we were always going to the chiropractor. We were doing the opposite of 'do nothing.' If you are doing, you have to do more. So we had to do something more: we discovered truck brake shoes. These work by pneumatic compression. Their compression gives the pressure to press down and release. Bob Kennedy was a genius. He put truck brake shoe mechanisms into the rice cake machines; soon he had all automatic rice cake machines. Now they have many machines: rice goes in, press down and release, cakes come out – all automatic now. So no more shoulder breaking. And workers are doing nothing. They reached the level of Lao Tsu.

Chico San was not so easy to build up. I understand Chico San just started making money last year. There was a fire several years ago; when we first started to make miso, we had 200 kegs of miso and a rice cake machine started a fire. The whole factory went up. We lost the factory. So Chico San started from scratch again. That is the history of Chico San.

For the Foundation, after Lou Oles took over he moved to Los Angeles and started the Ohsawa Foundation with the help of Jacques de Langre. Unfortunately Lou became very sick; he had cancer before macrobiotics, and he thought macrobiotics seemed to cure it. But it wasn't cured completely. When he learned that Ohsawa died, Lou somehow lost his strong leadership and started going off the diet. He often went to restaurants. His cancer started again; when he realized, it was very severe. He thought nobody could help, so he decided to go to Japan. He tried to ask for help in Japan but he was too late . . . he died over there.

Mrs. Ohsawa asked me to continue the Ohsawa Foundation, so I took over. Mrs. Oles and I continued. At that time I was living in Carmichael, near Sacramento, and I started a lecture trip of the entire U.S. At the end of the lecture trip (1970) I went to Mendocino County – John Deming asked me to stop over. He asked me, please come to my property; he had 60 acres in Mirimichi. He asked me to take this land. He wanted to give it to me. My wife didn't want it, but finally we decided we would receive this gift. That was the first macrobiotic resort, in Mendocino county. Later on I found out the reason he rushed to give it to me: otherwise, he would have paid $1,000 in taxes. It was a very nice piece of land, but I couldn't have the Foundation there; too wet, and other drawbacks. Later I sold it.

Then I moved to San Francisco, around 1971. At that time, many hippies were living in San Francisco. A new scene started for macrobiotics. About hippies, Peter knows very well, so now we hear from Peter. Thank you very much.

May 1972

George Ohsawa Seventh Year Memorial Ceremony

This is the seventh year since George Ohsawa left this world. Each year since his death I had hoped to have a memorial ceremony honoring his life and teachings, but it has never been realized until this year. The first memorial ceremony for Ohsawa in America was held at the Gedatsu Church of San Francisco on April 16th, conducted by Archbishop Eizan Kishida. It was a beautiful spring day of happiness and we gathered to give appreciation to our teacher Ohsawa and to renew our gratitude for the importance of his teachings.

There are several reasons why I chose the Gedatsu Church in San Francisco as the place for the ceremony and asked Archbishop Kishida to conduct the ceremony.

First, Ohsawa gave a lecture on macrobiotics at this church in 1963 by invitation of Mr. Koda, founder of Koda Rice Farm in California. Ohsawa met Mr. Kishida at this time and was impressed by Kishida's good physical and spiritual character. After the meeting he said to me, "You must keep in contact with him." Therefore, I visited Mr. Kishida as soon as I moved to San Francisco last year and at that time I became a member of the church.

Second, the doctrine of the church is based on Shinto, Taoism, Confucianism, and Buddhism, which are the foundation of Ohsawa's teaching. Gedatsu Kongo, the founder of the church, taught the importance of the Brown Rice Shrines at Ise which honor grains as a deity, saying that all races should realize their importance. It is no wonder that Archbishop Kishida, at present the highest leader of the Gedatsu Church of America, advises the macrobiotic diet to the members.

Third, the Gedatsu Church and Ohsawa teach basically the same way of life because both teach the importance of appreciation, no waste, understanding of wisdom, detachment from ego desire, and humility. They differ mostly in the usage of words and how the principle is applied in life. Both teachings have advantages and shortcomings. Someone who has not achieved happiness through macrobiotics may benefit and discover happiness by the teachings of the church. These are the reasons I chose the church as the place for the ceremony.

After the ceremony, a party was held and several people who had luckily met Ohsawa spoke, giving their impressions of him and his teachings. These, of course, did not give us the whole picture of Ohsawa, but gave some glimpses to those who unfortunately missed meeting him.

I would like to add my view about him here; that is to say, what was the most important teaching of Ohsawa. Someone will say it is the diet, some will say the order of the universe, and others will say appreciation. These are all correct, if you become happy by those learnings. In other words, the most important teaching is that which makes you most happy anytime and anywhere. One must choose the teaching or teachings from many which help him to be happy. Therefore, there are few teachings, if any, which are good for everyone. The most important teaching of Ohsawa for everyone, it seems to me, is to give.

Many macrobiotic students are not happy even though they have improved their physical condition very well. The reason for this is they don't give enough. They take in more than they give. They eat more than they can use or digest. They have learned yin and yang more than they can apply in daily life.

Ohsawa considered Lao Tsu as the freest man. Lao Tsu said in the *Tao Te Ching,* Chapter 48, "One who studies intellectually increases knowledge every day. However, one who studies Tao decreases what he has (such as ego-desire, ego-idea, and ego-clinging) and finally reaches *wu wei* or Nature. Nature just gives. One who gives always accomplishes everything because he is Nature."

Ohsawa taught to give, but he also taught what to take (eat). Lao Tsu taught only to give. Who was wiser?

In my opinion, Lao Tsu was wiser, but Ohsawa was kinder.

Never Mind vs. No Matter

What is mind?
No Matter!
What is matter?
Never Mind!

Time Magazine

When I first came to America, one of the many expressions I could not understand was 'never mind.' After being here ten years, I realize at last that it sums up the thinking of most Americans. This is the country of 'never mind.'

The strongest motivation in American life is a 'matter' called money. Many fortunate people, after immigrating here, found much of this matter and enjoyed a life of pleasure. Because of our great wealth of resources, the idea developed that everyone is entitled to such matter. This attracted people, most of them with only sensory or sentimental judgment. Since the average person reacts in a preconditioned or emotional way, the money-maker or the adventurer has become a hero in this country.

As a result, how to make money or how to achieve comfort and pleasure is the principal aim of our education.

By contrast, 'no matter' is the characteristic concept of the people of the Orient. Their education aimed, originally, at reaching highest judgment – *satori* – through an understanding of the order of the universe. This idea prevailed until

Western civilization – a materialistic, scientific technology – was imported.

Ninety years ago, the Japanese people used beautiful wood-block prints as wrapping paper for exported goods. This shocked Europeans who admired the paper as much as the commodities wrapped in it. The Japanese, however, had a different scale of values, not a lack of appreciation for art. They knew the instability of this world – the young become old, beauty fades away. That is why they called woodblock prints "pictures of the floating world." To them, material things, however beautiful, did not 'matter.'

At about the same time in France, Pasteur discovered a technique which would preserve wine and beer (*Etudes sur la Biere,* 1877). In his honor, the method was called pasteurization. A similar technique had already been used for several hundred years in Japan in the brewing of rice wine (sake). The inventor, however, has been forgotten. There is no record of his name. Why?

Not many years ago, the Englishman Fleming accidentally discovered the penicillium mold in his laboratory and observed that it destroyed bacteria. From this, penicillin was produced. It was called the "wonder drug" and has had so much influence that a whole series of drugs called antibiotics has resulted from it. This very same penicillium had been used in the production of dried bonita (Japanese fish) for hundreds of years before Fleming. Yet, no one knows who originated the idea. Why?

The reason is simple. The ancient Orientals didn't care or 'mind' about a material discovery, however useful it might have been. They only cared or minded about teaching life, highest judgment, or *satori* (in the Zen school). They admired only those who taught *satori,* the way of Zen, or *nirvana.*

This difference of viewpoint has produced two entirely different civilizations – the East and the West.

Conclusion: Science has studied matter and reached 'no

matter.' Religion has taught mind and has met 'never mind.'

The Westerner will not say 'never mind' and cancel an H-bomb test. The Oriental will, for he knows the order of the universe. "Everything that has a beginning has an end." Civilization began and therefore it will end, sooner or later. Never mind. Our true Real Life in Infinity will go on.

Destructive, analytical Western thinkers must learn from the ages-old, constructive, panoramic, Oriental mind – for our world teeters on the brink of self-destruction. Life could disappear in a flash.

This is literally a case of no matter.

Macrobiotic Principles

More important for your well being than diet is your attitude – how you feel about yourself, how wonderful life is, how amazing the snow and sun. You should have this feeling every day. Understanding yin and yang is also important but you must start with this feeling of wonderment.

The Here and Now of Eating

In psychology, focusing on the here and now is a popular technique, but it is not applied to diet. Eating here and now is macrobiotic. If you eat summer foods in winter, your physical and psychological condition becomes off balance. Eating here and now means eating foods grown close to your living space. Your best food is grown in your backyard. In Japanese, the symbol for food for guests is *running*, meaning one runs back and forth from the garden with fresh, seasonal food for the guests.

Eat the Whole Cow

George Ohsawa advised eating only whole foods. If you eat meat, eat the whole cow from top to tail. Watch animals. They eat bones and guts, which provide plenty of alkalinity. That's why they don't suffer from acidity. Because you eat only part, you develop an acidic condition. If you eat shellfish, you should eat the shell. Since the shell is not digestible, you shouldn't eat much shellfish.

Fiber and Disease Prevention

What disease is most fatal in the U.S.? Heart disease. But scientists found no heart disease among primitive people in Africa. Their diet included much fiber, since they ate only whole foods. How does fiber prevent heart disease?

Doctors warn heart patients not to consume too much cholesterol. But this substance is produced by the liver and has an important function in digestion. When there is fiber in the diet, cholesterol changes to bile. Without fiber, the cholesterol doesn't change; it goes to the bloodstream and becomes deposited in the arteries, overworking the heart.

How amazing is the heart! It beats around 70 times a minute, 4,200 times an hour, 100,800 times a day, 36,792,000 times a year. We're so lazy in comparison. We rest and sleep. The heart has no resting time. Two billion beats in 50 years. Amazing. Compare the heart to a piston: What car lasts 50 years? To beat two billion times, the heart needs much oxygen. What supplies the heart with oxygen? Arterial blood. Excess cholesterol plus three poisons – refined grain, white sugar, and refined salt – produce heart attack. Doctors say eat bran for fiber. But if you eat whole food, there is no need for bran.

The biggest cancer in the U.S. is colon cancer. The high amount of roughage in whole foods helps prevent colon cancer. Without roughage, the liver bile produces two acids which have been linked to colon cancer (apcholic acid and methyl cholanthrene). In the presence of these acids, toxic bacteria profligate when food remains in the intestines three days or more. With roughage in the diet, no old food remains in the intestines and only beneficial bacteria live there.

No Flies in Our Outhouse

Visitors to Vega Institute are amazed when they see our compost-producing outhouse. There is no smell and, consequently, no flies – even though we use no chemical disinfectants. This is due to our diet, of course.

Doctors are just discovering that large feces are a sign of health. The term for large feces in Japanese is *big transportation* – from mouth to excretion. The term for urine is the opposite – *small transportation*. There is less urine when the kidneys are able to reabsorb fluids back into the bloodstream, so there is less loss of minerals. Modern civilization is the reverse – small bowels and much urine.

Macrobiotic people watch food very carefully but forget to watch what comes out. Watch what comes out and you'll find your balance. Heart attacks and cancer have a beginning. They may be found in the end.

The Abuse of Memory

I talked with a young macrobiotic student at a recent lecture. He was as dependent, dreamy, and lacking in practicality as when I had known him before. He had been asked to stay at the beautiful house of his father-in-law and work as a gardening helper. But the father wouldn't let him stay in his house because he made them nervous and did not follow instructions. This was a man who transmuted a jewel to a mudball. He made unhappiness from happiness. He was not grateful at all for the situation, jobs, and offers. Why was he not grateful? He thought his love for his wife was true love. In reality his love was the love of his ego, not of her. Therefore, his love caused exclusivity, frustration, nervousness, and unhappiness for all.

What is the cure of this ego desire? How can we be free from the rigidity of ego? A free man is a man who is free from a rigid ego. How can we achieve this?

He was intelligent and a good student of macrobiotics. He was happy and did a good job with his work. Then he met a nice girl whom he loved so much that she accepted his proposal of marriage. It was a happy marriage. There is yang (happiness) and there is yin (unhappiness) – it is so true. Their unhappiness grew in the middle of happiness. Since he loved her so much he wanted to protect her from the outside world (social affairs) or bad vibrations which he thought others would give her. He refused to let anyone talk to her,

45

even on the telephone. He confined her in their apartment. He escorted her every time she went out shopping. He became more and more exclusive. His diet became very exclusive – almost rice only. The result of such a mono-diet made his thinking and attitude more exclusive. She became unhappy, fearful, and nervous. She escaped into her parents' home, where he moved in too. He was too arrogant to accept his father-in-law's advice and criticism. He left their home and moved into a study house. What a miserable end of a happy marriage. Why did such unhappiness result from such original happiness? He had an image of an ideal marriage through macrobiotic learning. He tried to follow this idea rigidly and stubbornly. This fixed and rigid mind prevented him from thinking flexibly. He completely lost his flexibility. He cannot work at any job except odd jobs. He is not flexible enough to adapt to situations. Inflexibility stopped his transmutation. His blood stagnated. His metabolism slowed down. His ki energy did not flow.

Why did he become so rigid and inflexible?

I have met many good students of macrobiotics who had a similar problem. They knew macrobiotics very well in principle, as well as practical points. Since they knew it so well, they liked to lecture on macrobiotics, without exception. They could lecture because of their good memory of books, lectures, or writings. Since they had good memory they had no trouble in explaining macrobiotics even though they did not live their understanding.

To them, understanding and living are two different things. They thought they understood macrobiotics even though they were not living what they preached. Their understanding came not from living but from memories of reading and hearing about macrobiotics from Ohsawa and other leaders. Their unhappiness is caused by their good memory. Ohsawa said the fourth condition of health is having a good memory. I find that many American youths are suffering from good memory. Their good memory made it easy for them to study anything – even macrobiotics. They show good understanding superficially. They memorize the teaching so easily they do not need to think or to practice the teaching in their lives.

Their good memory made them brain workers instead of physical workers. They never learned to earn a living by sweat. This made them more yin – lazy. This laziness made them dependent. They think that physical work is an ignorant person's job. They are too smart to earn a living through physical work.

Good memory made them think they knew philosophy very well; arrogance followed.

One who has a good memory is a lucky man. As Ohsawa said, good memory is a sign of good health. However, American youth abuse it. One must use his physical body in the daytime and his brain at night. If he lives like this he may become a happy man.

I met a man such as this in Los Angeles. He wanted to be a macrobiotic leader. He studied macrobiotics in books and lectures. He filled his brain with many concepts and the ideas of others. One day he threw away all that garbage. He is living on his feet now. He is very happy with his wife and a daughter. He is a door-to-door salesman with great success and confidence. He doesn't bother with any idea or concept except his happy feeling.

This attitude toward living is not the best. After several years of such a job, more boredom will come. However, for the time being it is good for many intelligent American youths to live on their feet. It is a very healthy tendency that many young Americans are doing agricultural work. Concept and practice, idea and finance, thinking and doing must be balanced.

Another bad result of good memory is that one remembers mistakes and feels guilty for a long time. This can be a good thing, because this consciousness causes us to improve our character. But the long memory of a guilt complex or sadness is mental depression. After we once felt guilty, we better forget the sadness of it. However, many people remember the mistakes and suffer from the memory.

Such good memory does not help achieve happiness. Such good memory seems to me to be popular among meat eaters and less popular among vegetarians and grain eaters. In any case, there are few who have a good memory of their benefactors. Most people easily forget benefits they received but remember for a long time something they didn't like. One who has a good memory of his good fortune and gives thanks all the time is a happy man. One becomes unhappy if he is not thankful for his life even though he has a good memory.

Forgiveness and Marriage

Is Forgiveness a Virtue?

Hate, resentment, anger. Unfortunately, we have these things. However, we cannot stay in these states forever, because we suffer from such mental conditions. Therefore, we try to get out of these states to real love. If these feelings are suppressed, they cause real suffering. One way of getting out of hate, resentment, and anger is forgiveness. Forgiveness makes ease, comfort, and peace of mind. Therefore, many religions teach forgiveness as a virtue. True forgiveness is all-embracing love, and very difficult to attain. However, when people forgive, they usually do not forgive through true love; they are forgiving because they are taught to do so through Christianity or other ethics, or they are forgiving because they cannot stand hatred emotions. In other words, they are forgiving sentimentally and still carry some feelings of hatred or resentment deep in their minds.

Later this trace of resentment becomes bigger and bigger until one cannot control it. Then he cannot forgive because this time his emotion of hatred or resentment is his creation, and no one else's. Then he has to expose his emotion or leave his partner or friends.

Someone said to me on a summer lecture trip that forgiveness is the only valid teaching of Christianity. When I heard this I felt arrogance. Who can give forgiveness in a case of betrayal, or when his own child is kidnapped or something like that?

Many feel guilty when they cannot forgive others because of the strong influence of religious teachings. This is another shortcoming of the ethical teaching of forgiveness.

Why should we not express our hatred or resentment frankly when we have it? We should not pretend we don't have it. We show anger when we have anger. Then we do not hold back any trace of budding anger which grows bigger later. Therefore I say, don't forgive when you can't really forgive from your heart, so that you have a chance to reach real, embracing love.

Why Do We Have So Many Marriage Troubles?

A friend of mine in Miami asked me this summer, "Why do macrobiotic people have so many marriage troubles?" In fact, I heard that six macrobiotic couples have been divorced or separated recently. Should not macrobiotic living solve marriage troubles?

In order to continue to have a happy marriage, we have to improve ourselves in the following ways:

– Man and woman must be equally healthy physically and should have an evenly balanced sex appetite. In other words, they must be yang. A macrobiotic diet will improve this eventually. Therefore, this is not the problem.

– A husband must be able to support his family financially and the wife must maintain an orderly home. To do this, they have to work hard. They must be yang. Lack of this hardworking, yang quality may cause a short-lived marriage because working hard (yang) brings a family or husband and wife together. When they are not working, the marriage may disintegrate due to the lack of a yang, centripetal force.

– In order to keep a marriage, not only do we need yang but yin also. One yin quality is patience. Marriage requires much patience. Without patience and endurance one cannot overcome the problems, difficulties, emotional stress, or differences in opinions that a husband and wife have. Men or women who are too yang often lack patience. They marry in a hurry and separate in a hurry. I have seen many American women who have hair on their legs or arms. This is a result of eating too much animal foods; they are too yang. No wonder there are so many divorces or separations.

– The last and most important quality which makes a marriage last a long time is the attitude: try to be loved. When first married, any husband and wife will love each other. And soon they separate. Their love doesn't last. Why? It seems to me they are not trying hard enough to be loved. Our love is quite egoistic and sentimental, relative. Our love can easily be lost when we see other women or men who seem to be more kind or beautiful.

We cannot expect his or her love to be perfect or eternal; we can only expect our own love to be perfect and eternal. For this we have to try to be loved. A man's talent or fortune may attract women for a while but it will not last long if he does not try to be loved. Once we try hard to be loved, then our husband or wife will love us for a long time. No husband can love his wife more than ten years for her beauty alone. However, he will love her for his whole life if she tries hard to be loved, even if she is ugly. There is no love in this relative world without the effort to be loved. There is true marriage when a husband and wife try to be loved.

Macrobiotics and EST

In San Francisco, Seattle, and Boston – many macrobiotic students are taking the EST training. Someone asked me why this is so. The reason is simple. They are not happy by macrobiotic learning. Why? Because they use macrobiotics as an excuse for their mistakes, failures, or wrongdoing. For example, when they fail to come to work at a promised time, they use the excuse that they ate too much yin food or drank too much beer the night before. They attribute the cause of laziness to the food they ate and not themselves. They refuse to take responsibility for their failures or mistakes.

One time one of the Foundation workers made a mistake by pasting up the magazine by odd pages on the left side of the book. When I asked him why he made such a mistake, he said he ate too much. For him, macrobiotics is a tool to make excuses. When one excuses his failures or mistakes, he never learns by his mistakes and he stays dumb as before. Because he makes excuses, others lose close interest in him. By excuses, he feels good and he stays a good and capable man, but gradually people leave him alone. He is too wise to be advised. If he admits that he is wrong, he feels miserable for a while, but he gains friendship, help, and togetherness. Often, mistakes and failures make real friends if someone is humble.

One who makes excuses or escapes from responsibility is not humble. One who is not humble cannot be loved. One who is not loved is unhappy.

52

One who uses macrobiotics as a tool to excuse his wrong-doings can never be loved and he is unhappy. As a result, he seeks other teachings. EST teaches that everything you are or do is your responsibility but not food. Then macrobiotic students begin to stop making excuses based on food. This makes their life happier. This is one of the reasons many macrobiotic followers are taking the EST training. However, if one takes EST training as a tool to excuse his wrongdoing, then he stays unhappy.

Whether he is happy or not depends on how he thought, how he behaved, how he ate, but not what he learned. Until he becomes a humble, honest, and lovable person, he is never happy, whether he is a macrobiotic, EST, Zen, or Yoga student. There are many roads to follow to reach happiness or freedom. Whatever method you may choose, if you stick to it long enough you will have much development in life as long as you avoid chemicals in foods and too many refined foods.

East West Journal Interview

EWJ: What is your view of the current variety in sexual life-styles – gay, celibate, androgynous, group, etc.?

HA: Everything in the universe is always in a state of change – from slow to fast, cold to hot, complex to simple, yin to yang, or vice versa. The present variety of sexual life-styles is only one example of a general tendency in our present world toward yin: complexity and variety, moving eventually toward dissolution. Our diet is also becoming more yin: diverse, highly refined, away from simplicity. Even the weather seems to be changing in that direction, with colder winters and greater temperature ranges. Not only are sexual lifestyles more varied, but the attitudes toward them are also looser, more relaxed, gentle – in other words, more yin.

Gay and the other sexual lifestyles you mention have existed since ancient times here and there among certain classes of society and in certain parts of the world which have special environments, diets, or general lifestyles favoring the development of these sexual orientations. However, it seems that these sexual lifestyles have become more common recently. I think there are several causes for this, of which the major one is our modern diet.

In particular, our large consumption of refined sugar tends to stimulate an increased secretion of female hormones in both sexes. The accelerated intake of chemicals – whether as food additives or as fertilizers and pesticides in the growing of food – affects the functioning of the glandular and nervous systems.

This variety may have a disruptive effect on society but it is itself a cause-and-effect manifestation of the laws of nature, whose orderliness is inescapable.

EWJ: What is the future of the family: nuclear, extended, other?

HA: Again, there's a trend toward variety, moving toward dissolution. Yang changes to yin and then back again. So there's also a minor current starting toward old-style families again. There are combinations of these two now. In one community called Synanon, where they help drug addicts and have a rather strict emphasis on discipline and things like that, their approach to the family is to take the children away from the parents after weaning. The group takes care of the children. There are advantages and disadvantages to that. I think eventually most people will turn back to what appears to be a natural tendency to want to take care of their own children. Of course, there are difficulties there too. Yin and yang work together. There's a back to every front. A close family may be good for children, but the important thing is for them to start going out on their own when they pass the age of twelve or thirteen.

EWJ: What is the best way to bring up children?

HA: The best way is sometimes the worst way. We think having only one parent – for example, after a divorce or death – is bad. But most great men lost one or even both parents when they were very young. They had to become independent. The writer Upton Sinclair, for instance, had a father who was a drunkard. Sinclair developed a burning sense of social justice. His life was dedicated to building a society that wouldn't produce drunkards.

In general, I think the most important influence on children is the mother. Up to the age of ten or eleven, they absorb her spirit; they watch her and imitate her ways. That's the basis of character. If the mother works very hard, the children acquire that habit; if she's very religious and humble they also tend that way. After ten or eleven years old, of course, they must begin to become independent of her.

EWJ: What makes a happy home?

HA: Many things, of course, but it is essential that at least one parent have high judgment. Then, whatever trouble comes along, they can find a solution. That keeps the family on keel.

EWJ: How do we prepare for a meaningful old age?

HA: It seems we start asking that question around the age of thirty. We should spend the years from twenty to thirty looking around, experimenting, travelling, trying everything, finding ourselves, discovering what we really want to do with our lives. Then around thirty we start working at that. For a meaningful old age, that work should be about 60 to 70 percent for personal satisfaction, and 40 or at least 30 percent to serve others, giving ourselves to people and society at large. If we don't, then our old age may be very lonely. You can't build a meaningful old age in one day.

August 1978

Honda

George Ohsawa defined happiness: "To do anything we want and enjoy it, day and night, up to the end of our life, realizing all our dreams and being loved by all during life and even after death. Such life is happiness itself."

Most of us are looking for what we want to do. We find a job that we want; later we find that job is not what we want. So we change the job. We find a mate we want; later we find he or she is not what we want. Separation or divorce follows. Our life is a continuous search for what we want.

Macrobiotics is a way of life which will help us find what we want and stick to it, day and night, to realize our wonderful dream and great joy.

There are many people who know what they want, and work hard for its realization. And many of them fail because they lose their health or make enemies along the way (too exclusive). Very few people have a dream that continues through their whole life. I found a man who had a lifelong dream. His name is Soichiro Honda, the creator of the Honda Motor Company. He did not know macrobiotics but he grew up in a natural macrobiotic way and at the age of sixteen he knew what his lifelong dream was.

Ohsawa said that school education dulls our intuition. Mr. Honda had only six years of schooling. He learned by working. Because he had no engineering training, his concept of engines and cars was not set by others. He could think freely.

As a young man he designed and manufactured a small- engine motorcycle and, later in his life, a compound vortex-controlled combustion engine.

Here is an excerpt from *Honda* by Sol Sander: "In the spring of 1974, Soichiro Honda – a man who managed to escape formal education more than most members of his generation and who has had a great deal of scorn for book learning – was given an honorary doctorate by Michigan Technological University. Honda talked simply and sincerely to his 'fellow graduates' on the occasion of the honor: 'Many people dream of the hope for success. To me, success can be achieved only through repeated failure and introspection. In fact, success represents only one percent of your work which results only from the ninety-nine percent that is called failure.' "

This is his conclusion after many years of trial and error to accomplish revolutionary motorcycle and car engines. In Honda's case, the object is a machine. When we want to improve our health, this need for hard work and constant trial and error is even more important. Good health is difficult to achieve. Even with macrobiotics, success in healing comes only after many failures.

It is common for people to give up macrobiotics when they fail to improve their health after a few months. This is mainly the result of their lack of strong understanding that one must look for the cause of the illness at its very root. Mr. Honda understood this completely and his success proves it. He said: "I wish to emphasize that the solution to any problem should be sought at its root. As as example, the air pollution problem. Automobile exhaust pollution is becoming a serious problem throughout the world. At Honda Motors we tackled the problem of how to clean exhaust gases within the engine itself. We knew that the basic solution could be achieved only if the exhaust gases were clean as they came out of the engine. We changed the combustion process itself and developed the CVCC engine system. The U.S. Environmental Protection

Agency found that this engine can meet the stringent emission standard of the Clean Air Act, without the use of after-treatment devices. This, I believe, is a success which could not have been achieved without a philosophy of seeking the solution of the problem at its root."

It is a pity that great car manufacturers like Ford and GMC don't change their attitude toward improvement of engines, even after seeing Honda's successes.

This need to search for the roots of problems is even more important in the medical field. It is clear that food is the source of our life. Therefore, if we seek better health and happiness we should study our diet. However, Western medicine today is interested only in the treatment of symptoms, mainly through surgery. Medical professionals not only ignore diet, they block development of a dietetic approach to healing. Macrobiotics and many other natural healing methods have been attacked as public enemies. But slowly, Western medicine is changing. For example, they now grudgingly admit the effectiveness of acupuncture although they still cannot comprehend why it works. Some doctors are also beginning to recognize the importance of diet in maintaining one's health. Their failure to find a magic cure for degenerative diseases – such as cancer, heart disease, diabetes, mental illness, etc. – has forced the medical profession to seek closer to the root of illness, which is diet. I believe that sooner or later some of the macrobiotic leaders will be honored by the medical profession and the public as great saviors.

We can learn much from Mr. Honda, though he worked with engines and not the human body. At a celebration honoring Mr. Honda, Japanese Prince Takamatsu said: "It must be an extremely exacting task to invent or contrive something?" Honda's reply was an important part of his philosophy which he has grafted into the company he founded: "I don't really find it very exacting because I am doing what I like to do. As the proverb says, 'Love shortens distances.' A person who is trying to invent something new is enjoying himself although he may appear to others to be having a hard time."

Our tasks and difficulties are much greater than improving an engine. Therefore, our joy and happiness will be much greater than those realized by Mr. Honda. He realized his dreams. And his success came from his philosophy of life which is the same as that of George Ohsawa. We must work hard to realize our dreams, just as Mr. Honda did. We can realize a very large dream because we know the Unique Principle. But we must work hard.

Psychological Transmutation

When we can transmute the vegetable world to our animal world, cells, organs, hormone and nervous systems develop. If these systems maintain a fairly constant state, we call this health. In other words, health is the ability to maintain our organism, metabolism, and body fluids fairly constant – even in a 130 degree Fahrenheit environment (equator) or a -30 degree Fahrenheit temperature (Alaska). This physiological constancy (health) is the foundation of biological and physiological transmutation.

The capacity for biological and physiological transmutation, however, is not enough for man to be healthy. Man must be able to transmute emotion: hatred and exclusiveness to love and faith. This transmutation is accomplished through our all-embracing supreme judgment.

Then, what judgment governs biological and physiological transmutation? This is mechanical, blind judgment – the lowest judgment. When blind judgment is very clear and precise we will be able to maintain health, which will reveal supreme judgment. Lowest judgment and highest judgment are the front and back of the same Oneness. Macrobiotics may be said to be a way of life which strengthens and clarifies the lowest judgment. When we have a strong blind judgment (instinct) we will reveal supreme judgment, which is omnipresent. As long as we live we are performing biological and physiological transmutation, yet emotional transmutation is difficult. Why? It seems to me that our blind judgment is not clear enough.

How do we strengthen blind judgment? Try to keep the efficiency of your living very high (least intake and much giving). How do we reveal highest judgment? Exercise your emotional transmutation as much as you can.

Here is some advice on emotional transmutation:

There is a woman who resents the fact that people do not like her because she is very active, open, giving, and hardworking. They say she is too yang. How can she get out of the spotlight? My advice to such people is to let others do things to help them. In that way you can avoid being first.

Another trouble I heard about at our summer camp is a kind of hatred. I had similar problems. Many people came to my house and some of them were very lazy. My wife, Cornellia, had a hard time agreeing with these lazy people. She hated them and complained to me. So I told her, he is lazy; he is bringing laziness to my house so that another stroke of bad luck will be expelled. Such small bad luck maintains constant happiness in our house.

The *I Ching* tells us, don't try to be perfect. Perfection is a step toward falling (the creative principle). When I advised a person to go and teach, he told me, "I am not able to teach; I am making so many mistakes." I told him, "That is how you can teach; tell about your mistakes. That is teaching." People learn more from your mistakes than from your success stories.

Whenever you have trouble with someone, don't complain to anyone else but him. Direct talk is helpful in most cases. The direct talk, however, must be done in such a way that you can clear up misunderstanding, prejudices, or preconceived ideas about each other. If direct talk is too intense, you will gain nothing.

If someone will not agree with you, then you may be wrong. If you really understand and agree with this, you will have no difficulty with others.

A New Life

Towards the end of summer camp, a lady from South America came to me for a consultation. She said she had been vomiting foods after every meal for many years. With this sickness, of course, she was skinny, weak, and even desperate about her future. She was not alive but like a wax doll.

Her father dominated her family and asked her to stay with him all the time. She hated this and felt she had been in jail. She tried to escape from her father several times. She took sleeping pills. Of course, the sleeping pills only made her mentality worse, damaging her brain. She had hated her parents so much that she didn't eat what they ate. She grew up eating mainly eggs, cheese, and onions. Several months ago she learned macrobiotics but she ate a lot of sugary foods after beginning the diet.

Sugar made her physically weaker, desperate, and negative mentally. She lost hope in her life. As a last resort she came to our macrobiotic summer camp.

After her confession, she asked me what to do. In her case foods work slowly because she vomits what she eats. How can she cure her troubles?

It seems to me that the vomiting is caused by her nervous disorder, probably a parasympathetic nerve disorder. To cure this, she must establish peace of mind. I told her that she must throw away her hatred for her father. He acted brutally because he ate an overly yang diet (too much meat) which made him too concerned and worried about her virginity. He loves her and in order to become a happy girl, she has to thank her father for his love. She agreed. Her cheeks brightened and her eyes shone.

I assured her that her troubles will go away as long as she stays away from sugar and keeps a yang diet without animal foods. She smiled and gave me a kiss on my cheek. After supper of that day, I asked her whether or not she still vomits. She said yes. A few days later, she was helping in the kitchen for the first time at camp and she was dancing at the campfire. Her vomiting had stopped!

She was so happy at the end of camp. She started a new, happier life.

Friendship

A boy I have known for years came to Vega one day. Next day I went to our garden to work; he came later. A while later he started asking questions about Vega and macrobiotics. Since I was busy in my scheduled work, I gave short answers rather abruptly.

Next morning after breakfast, he asked me to talk. He asked me why I was angry at him in the garden yesterday. He was unhappy because of my attitude. He was quite serious and tense. I told him that I was angry toward him because he disturbed my scheduled work by asking a bunch of questions which could be brought up at a meeting time or at resting time. Since we knew each other so long he thought he could ask any questions at any time. In fact, I didn't have so many feelings of friendship. Now after I argued with him for several minutes I felt friendship very much. He is much closer than ever. We communicated. We are friends.

H_2 and O put together do not combine, but if an electric spark is given, they do combine and produce water. Our arguments are like an electric spark which combines a man and a man. This is more so in the case of a man and a woman. When they combine, many sparks are produced. Arguments or quarrels between a husband and a wife are nothing but a process toward unification of their relationship. The bigger the difference of their characters, the bigger the sparks and the unification. The relationship between George Ohsawa and Lima Ohsawa was like that. There were many sparks between them in their daily life. These sparks are called arguments, quarrels, or fighting between humans and are considered undesirable by many. However, if we consider these human affairs as natural phenomena, we must welcome them because these tense mutual reactions only make our relationship deeper and stronger. There are those sparks between nationalities and nations which cause war. War between India and Great Britain or Japan and America were like that. The wars made their relationship much deeper, and mutual understanding increased tremendously.

Let us make our arguments with friends ignition sparks toward mutual unification – love or friendship.

Transmuting Dislike to Like

There was a beautiful lady student of mine at Vega. One day she said to me, "I don't like him." I was shocked. What an ugly word the beautiful mouth could produce! Is this the case that yang produces yin or beauty produces ugliness? Is our life at the mercy of this unique law?

She has been a student of yoga which is, I understand, a study of unification in living. Then she is not practicing yoga, because she has dislikes. She is wanting to be a teacher of yoga. Then she must overcome this disliking. Otherwise, her yoga will be just an exercise but not a true yoga. It is a yoga of body without spirit.

There are many persons like this. How many have reached a spirit of "I never met a man I didn't like" (Will Rogers)? When we dislike something or someone, we are exclusive and unfree. Therefore, there is no peace. Ohsawa taught us we must reach a spirituality of no dislike.

Is there any way we can overcome disliking? It is easy to talk about All-Embracing Love, but it's hard to practice. I know two things we have to practice:

One, we must establish health. As long as we dislike something, we are not healthy. We dislike sickness, poverty, inflation, unemployment, madness, war, flood, fire, insects, bacteria, hatred, anger, etc. Then we are not healthy. When we like everything, then we are healthy. How to be healthy? First, yin yang balanced natural diet such as is taught in macrobiotics. Second, work hard. When we are physically balanced, we dislike less. When I was young, I disliked eggplant. Now I like it very much. I was too yin then. When I became more yang, I was attracted to the eggplant (yin).

Two, we must transmute dislike to like. Don't think disliking is something inevitable, an unchangeable thing. For example, if you don't like rice, study how to cook rice so that you get to like rice. If you don't like your disease, you must work it out until you like the disease. As soon as you like the disease, you are cured. To me, there is no other way of a true cure, even a macrobiotic diet.

Cornellia was in the hospital for three years. She, of course, disliked hospitals and her sickness. She said "I can cure my sickness and become happy if I can go home." I said, "No, if you are not happy in the hospital, you will not be happy at home. If you dislike your sickness, you will not cure your sickness." Then she started to like the hospital and the sickness. She was always smiling in the hospital after that. Her sickness was cured three months later.

If you don't like him, you must change yourself so that you like him. Usually, we don't like someone because he or she has some shortcoming of ours. Our shortcoming refuses to accept another's similar character. This is the feeling of dislike. Therefore, dislike is a symptom of our arrogance which refuses to recognize our shortcoming. When we transmute dislike to like, we are happier.

Maintenance of Karma

I observed the all grain diet, number 7, for one month this past December. Why? The unhappy situation of my family forced me to look at my own shortcomings much closer.

My daughter Marie has been plagued with psychological problems. She dropped out of school because of teasing from her classmates. She enrolled in adult school to finish her high school diploma, but dropped that too because of the embarrassment she felt when reading her reports in front of the students. She became so nervous on those days when she had to read her reports that twice she took sleeping pills to become sick.

In October 1976 she went to see a family counselor without telling me or my wife. We became worried as the evening wore on and there was no sign of Marie. We reported her disappearance to the police, and finally at 2 a.m. the police called to say she was at the station. She had been wandering the streets since 9:30 p.m. after returning by bus from Chico. She had left before, and was told by Corneliasan that the next time she left, she would not be allowed back home. After missing school and returning from Chico late, she thought she would not be allowed back home.

Corneliasan believes Marie's psychological problems are due to the spirit of my ex-wife, who committed suicide 27 years ago.

One day Corneliasan and I went to the Gedatsu Church

where we pray to various deities and ancestors. This particular day, she asked the young minister, Reverend Sebe of the esoteric Shingon sect, to do the special training, Go-Ho Training, where one holds an amulet and prays. This amulet has writings of various deities and symbols of yin and yang written in Chinese characters. Many trainers have had powerful experiences holding this amulet. Some will write or speak words delivered from spirits of deceased relatives.

Corneliasan had such an experience. She began to speak the words of my ex-wife. The spirit (my ex-wife) said she made a mistake committing suicide and she regretted her deed. She was jealous of my present wife and this resentment and jealousy was cursing Marie to make her commit suicide.

Being a civilized and educated man, I found this difficult to accept. I believed it to be Corneliasan's subconscious speaking, not a spirit. Corneliasan didn't think that way; she strongly believed in the existence of the spirit and its cursing ability. She wished to ease the spirit's resentment and jealousy through prayer. "I can't believe that," I said angrily. "She committed suicide because she couldn't get along with my stepmother. She was too introverted to express her difficulties. It was her fault for committing suicide. Why should we suffer as a result?"

The reverend then said to me, "You can criticize someone when they are alive, but you can't criticize someone when they're dead. Her suicide was partially a result of your character, which may be causing the problems of your daughter too. The spirit tells you that until you can self-reflect and change your character, the unhappiness of your family will remain unsolved." He went on to say, "Your parents may have acted badly and caused resentment in someone. Such resentment may be the cause of your unhappiness. You may not think this right. Why should you be responsible for your father's deeds? However, because you have similar traits, you perpetuate this resentment. Rather than apologize for your parents, apologize for yourself. You must change your own behavior. The cause of your unhappiness is in you, not in the spirits."

"That's true," I reflected. George Ohsawa had said the same thing.

I realized everything happening around me was my responsibility. My ex-wife's suicide was my responsibility. It was due to my ego, my lack of independence, and my lack of understanding her difficulties. Now I realize that as long as I have these shortcomings, I will cause bad karma upon my wife and daughter. I am the one who caused my wife and daughter's unhappiness. I have to change my own self. That is why I went on an all grain diet for one month.

It didn't change my shortcomings immediately, but it did point out a few things for me: (1) Eating only grains increased my appetite. I was always hungry. Grains are obviously more digestible than other foods. (2) My stomach condition improved but not my intestines. (3) It was easy to overcome binge cravings.

I will continue this karma maintenance until my wife and daughter are happy.

Lima-San

July 13, 1972, Ann Arbor, Michigan: At last we met Lima-san, who looked as young as she was seven years ago. I was happy to see her. It was so pleasant talking with Lima-san. She radiated health and happiness, a good example of macrobiotics. Her presence alone makes macrobiotics meaningful.

However, I felt something missing. That was Mr. Ohsawa. When I saw Ohsawa in America, Lima-san was there always. Ohsawa was very yang, like a ginseng root; a self-made man. Lima-san was a flower in a hot house. Therefore, they were a perfect combination.

Ohsawa often lectured about marriage and birth date. The complete opposite date (180 days difference) of birth will make the yin yang attraction so strong that it is difficult for such persons to divorce each other. He used their marriage as an example of such a strong tie which he attempted in vain to break.

Everyone laughed when Ohsawa said, "I tried many times to divorce Lima but I failed." Many people may think this is a joke. But this is not a joke. In reality, they had difficulties and troubles between them all the time.

Since Ohsawa loved gentle, able women, it was often gossiped or rumored that he had a personal relationship with a secretary or some other macrobiotic woman. Lima-san, being a woman, was often annoyed, and suffered with jealousy from such gossip. On one occasion Lima-san came to me to talk about such a rumor which made her discouraged and distrustful of Ohsawa.

Ohsawa wanted Lima-san to be a macrobiotic example. Therefore, he educated her very severely. Sometimes we felt that Ohsawa was too severe and we felt very sorry for Lima-san, who accepted faithfully all scoldings and training from Ohsawa.

Lima-san's feminine patience was a great help in Africa and India where Ohsawa suffered from a fatal disease. Without Lima, Ohsawa would not have survived in Africa. It is Lima-san's patience and love for Ohsawa that has inspired her to continue the macrobiotic movement in Japan and to visit the United States.

The happiness radiating from Lima-san gathered many macrobiotic seekers in Ann Arbor and Chicago where she gave cooking classes with the help of Katharine Tanaka, Nobuko Ujiie, and Cornellia. Her cooking was thorough and perfect and the taste was delicately balanced. Her dishes are really masterpieces.

All who met her were encouraged and assured with the macrobiotic way of life.

She left Chicago for Boston, promising that she will come back to the United States again. Those who missed seeing her and tasting her cooking this year must prepare to do so in the next year.

April 27, 1975 at Vega

George Ohsawa Ninth Memorial Day Prayer

Almond and plum trees have blossomed, and cherry is blossoming fully now. It is a beautiful day. Here it is beautiful.

I, the president of Vega Institute, sincerely state in front of Amaterasu Oomikami, Sukunahiko No Kami, and Okuni Nushi No Kami that we, the disciples of George Ohsawa, are gathered to invite the soul of George Ohsawa here on his 9th memorial day for us to reunite and enjoy a day with him.

The foods which are offered here are all produced by your omnipresent, omnipotent, and omniscient love. We are offering those foods in order to show our appreciation for your gifts to us and to share these with our teacher, George Ohsawa.

George Ohsawa, you taught us how wonderful life is and how to live happily. We are immensely indebted to your teaching. Therefore, on your memorial day, we are gathered to offer you our delicious foods to show our small appreciation. Please accept our offerings and enjoy with us today's lovely party like you did when you were with us 10 years ago.

Although you never talk to us now, we can still hear your voice. You never show us your face, but we can see you. We are with you all the time. As you taught us, when we are separated we are together forever. Your voice when you said there is no death is still in my ear. You taught us that man is happy. If not, it is his fault. On this special day, we recall your

74

teachings and we promise that we will continue to realize your teaching forever. Please lead us to be a man of courage and honesty like you were. Please inspire us to make a happy family, community, and world, overcoming and enjoying all challenges and antagonisms. We are proud of you and we are happy.

Sincerely,
Herman Aihara

September 3, 1975

Learning From Salmon

One day after coming back from Japan, I went to the Feather River. Salmon were jumping the swift current all over. Late summer sun hit on the shore and it was a hot day. Around noon all fishermen had left except me. I cast a line over the middle of the stream which brought back an abundance of line. I wanted to pick up a metal spoon at the end of the line, so I started to pull on it. One end of the line was tight, but I loosened it finally. I pulled it. All of a sudden the line started to move by itself upstream. A salmon was on the line. What a surprise. I had gotten a salmon. It was moving faster and faster upstream. I tried to tie the line to my reel in vain. The salmon pulled the line so hard that my fingers hurt. I called Joe, Fred, and Mr. Kurosawa but none answered. Then the line broke. The fish was gone into the depths of the river for his spawning.

What strength a salmon has after travelling through 200 miles of water from the ocean! They don't eat during this journey, though. I sat on the river bank and gave thought to life for a while.

Salmon spawn upriver and go down to the ocean where they grow to maturity. At maturity they swim up the river until they reach where they were born for the first and last time. There they give birth to their offspring, and then die.

They spend most of their life in an ocean which is comparable to our life after schooling. The life of salmon and that of humans may not be much different except in old age. The old age of humans is retirement, but that of salmon is most adventurous. He fights all struggles a river can bring to him – fighting with another preying fish, fisherman's hook, swift current, etc. He spends all this effort for his offspring. After laying eggs, he just dies. What a simple and pure life. What an understanding. He is like an enlightened man. What a dedication to his offspring. What an understanding of the order of the universe. Modern humans consider sex just for pleasure. Making children is only the unwanted side product of their pleasure and a hazardous thing in their life. This is all right. Man can do anything he wants to do.

What I learned from salmon is that they take the most adventurous trip at the end of life – when we humans are retiring from living activity, to live with social security or retirement insurance.

Man should make the biggest adventure at the end of his life. Otherwise his life will be less interesting than that of a salmon. I know such a man: George Ohsawa.

Why Do Salmon Go Upstream? I

George Ohsawa once told us a mysterious story of salmon that swim up the stream to the place where they were born. Since then, I have been fascinated by the nature of salmon. I went salmon fishing on several occasions, and observed his strong power to swim up the river to his birthplace over 200 miles from the ocean. Not only have I been fascinated by his nature, but I also wondered why and how salmon know and find their exact birthplace from 200 miles away or more.

The following answer I found recently in a book entitled *Water* by Rutherford Platt (Prentice-Hall, Inc.). He writes:

> The "inextricable" mystery of fish taking the right turns was solved by an experiment which needed no microscopes. The researchers caught a hundred salmon just above the fork of an important tributary. They were all tagged for identification and the olfactory organs in the noses of fifty of them were removed. All were then transported below the fork and released. Those with clear noses unfailingly made the right turn, [but] those without smell organs were utterly frustrated, and took the wrong turn as often as the right.
>
> How does a salmon remember the odor of its birthplace? . . . The salmon detect their personal odor molecules even as they are mingled in myriads of various odor particles, because the scent trail of a salmon carries the

smell of the infusions of organic matter where it was reared.

Inquiry into this subject started at spawning spots – in a hideout behind an island in a lake, behind a boulder, in a quiet spot of water under the bank of a stream, in pebbles of a clear flowing brook. The research students watched while the female spawned her eggs and the male spread his milt over them, and they became buried by sediments – and then in a few weeks the young fry popped out and the water teemed with them.

If the fish are netted as soon as born and transported to another stream, they are imprinted with the odor of the spot to which they are transferred – not that of the place of birth. In short, the memory of an odor is not genetic. They did not get it from their parents. It is imprinted *by what they eat* after birth when they are little fry.

This is not brain memory. It is molecular memory, an instinctive memory that resides in all the cells of the body, instilled by what the fish ate in its first weeks after being born. The wonderful memory is exerted by protein enzymes inside cells, and hormones that carry the "memory" in watery body fluids to activate organs and muscles.

This story reminds me of a story in Okakura's *Book of Tea*. According to Lu Wu, the mountain stream is the best; the river water and the spring water come next in the order of excellence.

Ancient people distinguished quality of water – whether it came from the mountain stream, river, or spring – by its smell. Today we can distinguish whether water comes from the city or mountain by its taste due to chemical additives. In ancient times, when there were no chemical additives, they also distinguished types of water by smell. If our sense of smell would be so keen as the salmon's or as our ancestors', we could avoid adding chemicals to drinking water and avoid environmental pollution of water.

To get back to salmon, now I understand how the salmon goes back to his birthplace. But then another question came to me. Why does the odor of the birthplace attract the mature salmon? Can you answer this question? I don't think science can solve this, just as it cannot provide the solutions to such questions as why we have cancer, heart attacks, etc., because science is for the question of *how* but not the question of *why*.

Those questions will be answered by the philosophy of life which is the principle of yin yang. Please try to solve this question so that you can understand the importance and power of the yin yang way of thinking, and furthermore, the wonderfulness of life itself.

Why Do Salmon Go Upstream? II

After I wrote the last article, I read the next chapter of the same book, *Water*. The chapter called 'Why Do Salmon Do It?' attracted my attention. To my surprise, Platt did not answer his own question; instead, he wrote what I said before: "All the elegant techniques of science cannot find the why of anything in life. They can detect chemical structures of molecules such as DNA and the way they act, but this does not tell why they are as they are. However, wonderful *laws of life* have been discovered, and organisms seem to make sense when we see them conforming to these laws."

Wonderful! Mr. Platt is writing with excellent rationalization. However, the following writing disappointed me. "The law that interests us here is the traditional one perceived by Charles Darwin: species were the result of survival by natural selection. In other words, salmon must have evolved from ancestors who survived by dint of overcoming the great physical barriers to breed far upstream."

Then he questions again, "Why?" He is a thinker. "But why did their ancestors have to take such energetic steps to survive? Why did they have to breed *upstream?* The answer is that they didn't have to. They could have turned the other way and vanished in anonymity among myriads of ocean fish. . . ."

Author Platt gave up on *why* at this point, so he doesn't think *why;* instead he thinks *how,* as almost all scientists do.

Platt speculates how salmon acquire the nature to spawn upstream. His conclusion is that during the million-years evolution of fish, salmon acquired genes which do not permit eggs to be fertilized in salt water. During the ice age, according to him, the mouths of rivers were filled with fresh water due to the melting ice. Therefore, the fresh water spawning places must have been plentiful along coastlines, and salmon didn't need to go upstream for spawning. However, as the shrinking glaciers drew back, salmon had to swim upstream to find spawning places. His explanation is very good; however, he doesn't explain why or how salmon acquired genes which do not permit eggs to be fertilized in salt water.

So far I have never read books or met a man who answered the question: Why do salmon go upstream to spawn? As I wrote previously, the scientist gave up the question and answered the question about *how* salmon go up the stream to spawn.

Isn't this a shortcoming of science, especially of medicine? Recently science in general, and medicine in particular, have achieved tremendous progress. However, their progress was in learning how but not in discovering why. Man knows how to visit outer space, or the moon; how to calculate faster than our brain or a Japanese abacus; how to transplant hearts, livers, kidneys, and how to cut out malignant tumors. They don't ask why we have cancer, heart attacks, and kidney failure in the first place. In other words, modern medicine uses symptomatic cures. It cannot eliminate any diseases. It only chases away symptoms, and the causes of the diseases remain. Therefore, the sick who are treated by symptomatic medicine will remain sick and suffer the same malady, or another, with worse conditions.

In order to solve problems of life such as heart attack or cancer, we have to ask why we have such sicknesses before we ask how to cure them. In order to answer the question why, we must know the law of life. We must know how life operates or is controlled. In other words, in order to answer why we develop cancer, we have to understand the principles of life, the constitution of life, or the order of the universe.

According to Oriental philosophy, life, nature, and the universe operate by two forces – yin and yang. Life is the fabric interwoven by two forces: expansion and contraction, shady side and sunny side, minus and plus, negative and positive, acid and alkaline, female and male, peace and war. The interplay between these two forces follows certain rules which are called the principles of life or the principles of the universe. If we look at the mysterious world of life through these principles, many wonders can be solved. Let me solve the mystery of salmon through the principle of yin yang.

First of all, in order to solve the question why salmon go upstream, we have to ask why baby salmon go downstream. There is an upstream; it follows that there is a downstream. Here you see yin and yang already. One is yin, the other yang. According to the yin yang principle, yin attracts yang and yang attracts yin. This law is valid in all phenomena – in physics, chemistry, nutrition, medicine, economics, politics, marriage, and everything you can imagine. This law solves the mystery of salmon. Now you have to decide about a few things using yin and yang. Are baby salmon yin or yang? Is upstream yin or yang? Is the ocean yin or yang? Are salmon in the ocean yin or yang? Is a salmon egg yin or yang? When these questions are properly answered, the mystery of salmon is solved by simple logic.

First, think of salmon eggs, which are called caviar. This is a delicacy, served in high-class restaurants, which is round, red, compact, and salty. Therefore, it is yang. It is so yang that it rejects the ocean, which is also yang (salty, moving all the time); likes repel one another. Salmon have to find yin places to expel their eggs. This is the reason they go upstream, where the environment is yin – cold, quiet, and high altitude. The baby salmon which come out from the yang eggs are yin, although they have yang potentiality or inner yang character.

The yin baby salmon are attracted to the yang ocean; therefore, they travel downstream towards the ocean which is yang. The yin baby salmon overcome many difficulties in the river before finally reaching the ocean. This means they have become quite yang by this time, and that the weaker (more yin) salmon would have been eliminated in the journey downstream. The remaining salmon would grow in the ocean until mature. The cold water, powerful waves, attacks from bigger fish, storms and other such natural conditions with which the growing salmon must contend make them strong and yang. In four years, salmon become so yang that they are attracted to the yin, quiet, high mountain water. The yin place which attracts them most is their original habitat. Fragrances from their birthplace, the odor of foods, configurations and textures of pebbles, trees, and water are all lodged in their memory and exert a strong attractive power. Their inner instinct guides them to that place where they can bury their eggs.

During this journey they fast, and become even more yang, which intensifies their attraction to the yin upper stream. Once they reach their destination they happily lay their eggs, again being motivated by the natural forces of yin and yang. Yielding their most yang quality, eggs, the salmon become yin, lose their scales, lie on the bottom of the river, and finally disappear into the water.

So, the life of salmon is a typical example of yin yang phenomena. Please contemplate it. Isn't our life like this? Macrobiotically speaking, salmon is one of the most yang foods, and it is so delicious! Grilled, pan fried, or baked, it will make an excellent meal when served with radish, ginger, or lemon. Salmon bought in a store is usually less tasty because it is old. If you catch it in the ocean or a stream, the taste will be unforgettable.

Chewing is to Return
to God

One day a student at Vega asked me why we have lost the ability to select good food naturally anymore, and like to binge so much that we have to decide what foods to eat intellectually (such as using the yin yang concept). When people were eating good foods in ancient times, they must have had good judgment to select good foods from bad ones, relatively speaking. Why did they start to eat badly when they had high judgment?

I answered as follows:

In ancient times, foods were grown in nearby surroundings and in season. Therefore, whatever they ate was in good order. This improved or maintained their ability to select good foods on the intuitive level but decreased some ability on the conscious level because they didn't need to think about which foods were good for them.

Then food commerce developed. Foods were transported in distance (out of order in space) and out of season foods were supplied abundantly due to the development of refrigeration and hothouses (out of order in time). Industry made foods more out of order. Preservatives were added to prolong shelf life and prevent spoiling. Coloring and other chemicals were added to keep foods looking fresh, soft, and delicious on the surface. Fertilizers and insect control chemicals were used more and more in farming so that farmers would not lose any money in case of a bad harvest, and to make more profit. As a result, there are no more natural foods in our modern society.

Also, as a result, we lost the good judgment to select good foods even on the intuitive level. You may have experienced or known someone who could not stop eating sugary foods even though he is so yin that you think he should not need sugar. His judging ability to select good foods is clouded or distorted. Therefore, the study of nutrition has been developed and a concept such as yin and yang has been applied in the selection of foods. However, these are all in the intellectual level of our judgment. When our intuitive level of judgment is clouded or distorted, we may have big trouble in selecting foods due to strong cravings or the desire to binge. In order to improve our ability to select good foods intuitively, we have to continue eating good foods for quite a period of time. In other words, to continue eating good foods we need good intuitive judgment. This is a vicious cycle.

To me, there is only one other way to improve our judgment. That is chewing. Chewing well can give us a selective judgment of foods, consciously as well as subconsciously. By chewing, foods are liquefied. This is very important because in digestion, chemical reaction takes place in liquid form. If we chew well, foods are liquefied with saliva, causing chemical reactions in the taste buds, and we can judge if food is salty or sweet, bitter or sour, etc. If we don't chew well, only the surface is broken down and foods are only partially tasted. When we chew well, all the food is liquefied and we taste the whole food. When we taste the whole food, we can distinguish natural from artificial or chemically treated foods. When chewing well, synthetic chemical additives don't make a good taste – but natural foods will be tastier when chewed more. The macrobiotic diet, to me, is to eat foods which become sweeter and more delicious when we chew more.

The importance of chewing doesn't stop here. Chewing is a meditation and chanting without words. When chewing, our subconscious is occupied with the chewing action as happens when chanting. This brings consciousness out of the control of the subconscious. (Our consciousness is influenced by the subconscious most of the time.) When consciousness, which is our ego function, is free from the subconscious function, we have a great chance for contact with cosmic or universal consciousness which is enlightenment or satori. Chewing well is returning to God. Ancient Japanese had the same idea when they made the word chew. *Kamu* in Japanese means to chew, and *kami* is God.

When people made a habit of chewing less and eating in a hurry, they started eating badly even though they had good judgment on the intuitive level.

Eyes Lie Horizontally, Nose Lies Vertically

About 750 years ago, Japan had several distinguished Buddhist monks. One of them was Dogen, the founder of the Soto Zen sect. He was born on January 2, 1200 to a noble family. At a young age he lost his parents. This shocked him so much that he lost interest in pursuing earthly desires such as fame, fortune, or status. At the age of 13, when he was staying at his uncle's home at Mt. Hiei where the famous temple Enryaku-ji is located, Dogen decided to become a monk. He studied Buddhism hard. He was soon puzzled by a question to which he could not find an answer from any teachers. The question was why one has to study hard when Buddhism teaches that man's nature is Buddhahood.

In order to solve this question, he left Mt. Hiei and went to the monastery of Kenninji and became the pupil of the master Myozen (1184-1225), who was a master of the Rinzai Zen sect and successor of Eisai. Unable to satisfy his question, he asked the master permission to go to China with him. In spring of the year 1223 he left Japan accompanied by his master. They arrived at a Chinese port in the month of April. There he encountered his first lesson of Ch'an (Zen).

One day an old monk came aboard the boat on which Dogen was living, to buy mushrooms. He was a cook in a Zen monastery. Dogen asked him to stay on the boat for dinner to talk with him about Zen, but the old monk refused Dogen's proposal, saying he had to cook tomorrow's meal at the mon-

astery and he didn't want to lose his opportunity to cook because cooking was his study. Puzzled with the answer, Dogen
asked him with a superior attitude, "Cooking, you say, is your
study? Why do you not devote yourself to meditation or to
the study of books? Why do you think cooking is so important?"

The old monk laughed at him and said, "Oh, you young
foreign student, it is regrettable that you do not understand
what study is. If you want to know the answer, please stop
over at my temple. I will tell you."

Here Dogen got another question: "What is the Buddhist's
study?" In order to solve this question, he visited several
masters. During his pilgrimage, he mastered the school of
Ts'o Tung (Soto Zen) from the master Ju Ching. He stayed
for two more years with Ju Ching and returned alone to Japan
in 1227. When he returned from China, he brought back nothing, contrary to the customary practice of the Buddhist who
ordinarily returns from China with a load of sutras and sacred
objects. Instead he said, "I learned in China nothing but one
thing; that is to say, 'Eyes are horizontal and nose is vertical.'"

Many attempts to explain this saying have been made.
Here is my explanation:

His saying is the answer to the question, 'What is the Buddha Nature?' 'Eyes are horizontal and nose is vertical' is the
Buddha Nature, or, more precisely speaking, is a manifestation of the Buddha Nature. The study of Buddhism is to
realize this fact – that we all have Buddha Nature or that we
are all nothing but Buddha Nature. From the point of view of
the macrobiotic principle, the horizontal position is yang and
the vertical position is yin. Therefore, he is saying that our
body is manifested by yin and yang. In other words, Buddha
Nature is manifested by yin and yang phenomena or forces.
Buddha Nature is Tao, which is Nature's ultimate, and is
manifested by yin and yang, according to the teachings of
Lao Tsu.

Many scholars say that Ch'an (Chinese Zen) is influenced by Taoism. Therefore, it is not strange to assume that Dogen was influenced by Taoism too. If this is the case, his saying is the esoteric expression of the yin yang principle. Such esoteric expressions of yin and yang exist in all ancient religions or myths. For example, Buddhism has the bent cross, Christianity has the cross, Judaism has the crossed triangles, and Taoism has *tomoe* (the yin yang symbol).

What Dogen also brought back to Japan was his answer to the question the monk had asked when they were on the boat when he first arrived in China. His answer was that everyday living is the Buddhist's study. This is the basic principle of the Zen school which emphasizes the importance of everyday practice over the mental search for inner illumination. It is this practicality of Zen that explains why vast numbers of intellectuals, artists, and businessmen, as well as politicians of Japan, have been attracted to Zen. The practicality of Zen is well written in the excellent book by Robert Linssen, *Zen, The Art of Life* (Grove Press). According to Linssen, "Zen demands that we give great intensity of attention to anything we undertake. Reality is where we are from moment to moment. The factor determining our own realization depends on the mental attitude with which we confront our daily work and leisure. The type of work is secondary, for each incident and perception that we experience could be an occasion for Satori."

Therefore, when Dogen brought back the spirit of Zen from China, all the cultures of Japan were influenced by Zen. Linssen explains this: "The spirituality of Zen is expressed practically through different arts such as flower arranging, Japanese gardens, and paintings, as well as through fencing, judo, aikido, and also through customs, like the tea ceremony." Linssen states, "To understand the psychological origins of judo and aikido and their relations to Zen and Taoism, it is worthwhile to recall that the spiritual life of the Japanese people has been strongly influenced by the Chinese philosophies, and Ch'an in particular." The following aphorisms of Lao Tsu will help the reader to feel the mood of the *Tao Te Ching*, which inspired the masters of judo and aikido:

- Softness triumphs over hardness, feebleness
  triumphs over strength.
- That which is more malleable is superior
  to that which is immovable.

In conclusion, Dogen was a unifier of Buddhism and Taoism and this unification is manifested in all Japanese art and in all ways of life in Japan. One such way of life is Japanese or Oriental medicine. One of its arts is the Do of Cooking – macrobiotic cooking. As students of macrobiotics we have as our teachers Lao Tsu, Buddha, Dogen, and other Zen Buddhists. They are the masters who posed the questions that teach us the true spirit of macrobiotics. From their teachings came the basic foundation of the macrobiotic way of life.

The way one chooses to achieve or reveal his Buddha Nature is Tao, which is in turn manifested by yin and yang forces. Therefore, Oriental medicine aims to cure sickness and to reveal one's Buddha Nature – a man whose life manifests love, freedom, and justice. By the same token, through the art of cooking one attains the biological and physiological realization of Buddha's Nature. This type of cooking is far more than a mere technique aiming at better taste; it is an art which manifests the expressions of love, freedom, and justice through the forces of yin and yang in food.

Editorial

Not only America but the world situation is going mad and insane now. Describing two tragic situations in a recent issue of the *San Francisco Examiner* (July 14, 1968), Irving Bengelsdorf said that paradoxically, while the Ford and Rockefeller Foundations were cooperating in a program at the International Rice Research Institute (Los Banos, the Phillipines) to try and find new strains of high-yield rice to alleviate hunger in the Asian countries, the Air Force was busily destroying Asian rice crops by spraying herbicides containing arsenic on rice paddies in South Vietnam. Still more tragic is that both North and South Vietnam have populations of around 20 million, are considered poor and under-developed nations, and yet are not starving. South Vietnam could even afford to export millions of tons of rice per year. However, in 1964, due to general hostilites, many rice paddies were laid waste or made useless in South Vietnam. Now the United States exports about 600 tons of rice per year to South Vietnam. No one can even speculate what the long-term damage will be to the foliage, shrubs, and trees long after the enemy has been denied cover.

Why does America starve the noncombat people of South Vietnam, and not North Vietnam? Does a developed country mean hypo-rationalism? No, it means hyper-rationalism. As Mr. Bengelsdorf further points out in his article, the Defense Department, reacting to mounting scientific criticism, awarded $60,000 to the Midwest Research Institute in Kansas City to find out just what were the effects of herbicides. Benglesdorf reports Dr. Arthur W. Galton, professor of biology at Yale, as saying that much study concerning the ecological consequences of herbicide use, particularly heavy application, is factually deficient.

Another example of hyper-rationalism in modern civilization is CBW: chemical biological warfare. *Time* magazine reported (September 6, 1968) that the potential of CBW is being explored from the United States to Taiwan; the busiest in the field may be the Soviet scientists. Many books concerning CBW have been recently published. *Unless Peace Comes* (Viking), written by sixteen scientists and scholars from six different countries, warns about CBW, saying an entire population could theoretically be sent 'tripping' with a few pounds of LSD in the water supply. In *The Biological Time Bomb* (World), British science writer Gordon Rattray Taylor is concerned about genetic warfare – one nation permanently weakening the people of another by infecting them with potent lab-made viruses carrying hereditarily damaging material.

There will be no safe place on the earth in the near future. There are only two choices we can make: (1) evacuate to Mars or another planet! or (2) stop this confused civilization and change it to a new one. Escape from Earth is of no use. Man will repeat the same unhappiness. So long as his high judgment stays veiled, his low judgment will cause fear and protection devices (the 'armor' of Wilhelm Reich).

Many socialists envisioned a new society by adopting social reforms. Thomas Moore, Robert Owen, Karl Marx, Nikolai Lenin, Charles Fourier, Saint-Simon, Mohandas Gandhi, and Mao Tse Tung are some of the famous social reformers. Modern Russia, America, China, and India are the result of such social reforms. However, all nations are ever increasing in fear, disease, uncertainty, conflict, poverty, crime, killing, war, segregation, and hatred. Many scientists and scholars are trying to find solutions for these problems.

In *The Direction of Human Development* (Hawthorn), Ashley Montagu declared: "At the present time the greatest obstacle in the path of human progress is not the atom or hydrogen bomb or any other external obstacle, but in the disordered selves of human beings. Man requires no supernatural sanctions for love. Love is a fact of nature, and it is the most important of all the facts about nature. Love is and should be the most natural of religions for human beings. The person who has been brought up to be a loving human being will not be able to see the world in anything but loving terms. Violence will be as foreign to his nature as it is at present common to the acquired nature of most men of contemporary Western civilization. To most persons, conditioned as they are in the Western world today, love and violence are not only not incompatible but are perfectly reconcilable forms of conduct, whereas, in fact, violence is not only contrary to man's basic nature but inimical to it."

Montagu is correct in saying that love is a fact of nature. But it does not have much power to solve the present violence and disorderliness in the world. Why? Because he confuses supreme love with sensorial and sentimental love. The sentimental love for self or our own race will produce hatred of others. Mr. Ohsawa said this love is a synonym for hatred; friend is enemy. As long as we realize only sentimental or sensorial love, world violence will never cease.

How can we achieve supreme love? To me, all men live with supreme love but it is eclipsed by sensorial, sentimental love because the lower levels of love are more intense, stronger. Therefore, what we have to do is clarify supreme love from these lower levels of love by clearly understanding and distinguishing them. A clear distinction between lower and higher love is achieved by mental training, as many religious groups are doing. However, mental conditions are based on food. Diet must be given careful consideration. This is the reason many religions had commandments on diet.

According to our experience and other reports, meat is a food for violence. It is understandable why there is so much violence in this country, where the per capita meat consumption is one of the highest in the world. According to statistics, Americans consumed 163 pounds of cereals, 104 pounds of vegetables, and 214 pounds of meat per person during 1962. Moreover, some meat is "dead, dying, diseased and disabled," according to Ralph Nader, who candidly speaks out in *Playboy*, October 1968. What he says is shocking and much like *Jungle* by Upton Sinclair, published in 1906. "Mr. Nader said that the book (*Jungle*) helped bring about the Inspection Act of 1906, which called for the federal inspection of slaughterhouses. Today, however, conditions in much of the meat industry have worsened. The consumer cannot trust his senses because of 'chemical doctoring' and frozen storage, and consequently, he says, Americans are eating a great deal of bad meat." It is clear that eating such food causes not only individual disease but infects whole communities, making them fertile ground for riots, violent crimes, and mass fear.

Forever missing from the plans of all previous peace-seekers or Utopian architects is the consideration of daily food. Without changing the daily diet, America or for that matter the whole world will never find a safe place in the entire universe. We must become extinct. This does not mean that eating the proper food solves everything. I mean that eating the proper food helps us reach supreme love.

Eating properly does not always bring supreme love. We tend to be inconsiderate, jealous, hateful, and condemnatory even when eating well. We must admit these human weaknesses frankly and humbly. Only when we humbly admit our own smallness, exclusivity, sensorial and sentimental love can we admit and accept the smallness and exclusiveness of others. Therefore, we are able to embrace them. This is supreme love. We can never attain supreme love easily unless we discipline ourselves by proper diet and self-reflection (prayer). "Only the biological and physiological education of the constitution of the Infinite Universe can save man of his most serious disease: low judgment – which produces all disease, including thermonuclear war." (George Ohsawa, *The Atomic Age*.)

My sincere wish for all our friends is: After you establish your health, make your love go higher through humble reflection of your smallness, exclusivity, and sentimentality. Radiate your love (joy, confidence, inclusiveness) to as many people and as quickly as possible. Then we shall convince people the macrobiotic way of life brings peace in the world, a peace which will end the social revolution through individual revolution.

We now have a higher level revolution to perform in order to survive as man. This is the biggest difficulty humanity has ever had to meet. It is therefore our biggest joy, joining together to perform this honorable task.

Why Did Vietnam Win the War?

The North Vietnamese showed the world that a massive war machine, superior technical sophistication, massive firepower, billions of dollars spent on millions of pounds of bombs, defoliants, and napalm cannot destroy a tiny nation whose only weapons are brown rice and an intuitive understanding of yin and yang. We are discovering at the expense of many victims that power and force do not reign supreme in this universe. The Western military, like the giant Goliath, is big and cumbersome. An Oriental David, unprotected and unarmed save for a simple small sling and a few smooth stones, a supple and agile body, fearless spirit, and accurate aim, can overcome Goliath with all his armor and more sophisticated weaponry.

Flexibility, durability, supreme judging ability, intuition, and an ability to instantly adapt to change are the most formidable weapons. These capacities are the natural result of eating foods which create a flexible endurance – brown rice and vegetables.

Physiologically speaking, the Vietnamese must be very healthy because their sugar consumption is one of the lowest of the civilized countries.

According to nutritional theory, sugar is a nutritious food. However, our experience and that of many nutritional leaders has been strongly against this concept. Dr. John Yudkin, head of the nutrition department at London's Queen Elizabeth Hospital, one of England's top medical centers, told *The Enquirer:* "There is no doubt in my mind as to the link between sugar and serious disease. More and more scientists are beginning to agree that sugar is a causative agent in serious disease like coronary thrombosis and diabetes. . . . Refined sugar is so dangerous to health that its use should be restricted by law – like narcotics," says the leading physician and biochemist. "I would outlaw sugar completely, if necessary," he said. "Just as the law recognizes that cocaine is bad for you, the law should have something to say about sugar. . . . It's no good merely issuing warnings. The only result you would get if you told people that sugar could lead to death from a coronary is that they would say, 'Oh dear, what a pity,' as they reached for the sugar bowl."

Dr. Yudkin said he thought banning sugar production "would be more feasible than it sounds. You wouldn't have the bootlegging problems with sugar prohibition that were experienced with alcohol prohibition. It's relatively easy to make bathtub gin. But refining sugar is a highly sophisticated process that the backyard bootlegger couldn't possibly handle."

He said his conclusions about the dangers of refined sugar were drawn from extensive personal research on the relationship between diet and coronary heart disease. Refined sugar "was introduced into man's diet only 200 years ago," he said – at a time when coronary thrombosis was unknown. "Biologically, man has not had time to change into a sugar eater." But, he said, the average American consumes about 100 pounds of sugar a year – "25 times as much sugar in two weeks as our ancestors ate (in fruit and other natural forms) in a year."

"Sugar, like starch, is broken down by the liver which secretes cholesterol and triglycerides. These are fats which eventually form deposits around the heart and arteries. Sugar molecules are smaller than starch molecules and are broken down more easily by the liver. And because they are smaller, they turn into fat more quickly. There can be no doubt of the correlation between sugar consumption and a higher level of cholesterol and triglycerides."

"If we compare the diets of the well-off and the poor and set them alongside the statistics for heart disease, we find the wealthier countries consume more sugar and are prone to heart disease."

"There is no need for this sugar except for the pleasant taste we have become accustomed to." All the sugar actually needed by the human body can come from other food sources such as fruit, Dr. Yudkin explained.

He said as a first step in eliminating the problem he would suggest "a very heavy tax on sugar, as some countries impose on cigarettes. Even if that cut consumption by just three quarters or even half, it would be better than nothing."

The most important effect of sugar on physiology was shown in an experiment by a Japanese chemist, Dr. Chishima. According to Chishima, normal human red cells are destroyed by adding 0.9% sugar. Therefore, sugar is not only a robber of our nutrition, stealing vitamins, but actually a destroyer of our body. When red blood cells are destroyed, our nutritional needs will not be well supplied. Our immunization ability will be destroyed and therefore it is obvious that sugar eaters will be more vulnerable to disease than non-sugar eaters.

From the yin yang principle of macrobiotics, the danger of sugar was warned by Ohsawa for almost 50 years. He said sugar is 100 times more yin than water. Even by giving up only sugar, many sick people can improve immediately. There are no words to express the stupidity of a man who cannot give up the use of sugar.

I strongly believe that the following chart provides evidence as to why Vietnam won the war without using dreadful weapons against the world's strongest country, the United States.

Sugar Consumption per Capita per Year

Nation	1961 (lbs.)	1964 (lbs.)
North Vietnam	1.32	2.20
North Korea	3.96	3.96
South Korea	6.16	2.86
People's China	8.36	6.16
South Vietnam	9.90	10.12
Formosa	24.20	24.20
Japan	35.20	37.40
West Germany	70.40	72.60
USSR	81.40	79.20
USA	105.60	101.20
Switzerland	118.80	94.60
England	121.00	114.40
Denmark	123.20	121.00
Ireland	134.20	129.80

February 1974

Japanese Alphabets and Brain Functions

The Japanese believe that everything expresses itself by voice – even 'lifeless' things such as rivers, trees, and mountains. However, man is far superior in voice communication compared with other animals, plants, or things. Pavlov called words the second communication system, since he thought that shape and color are the first communication system. The second system requires a higher function of the brain than the first system. Therefore, it can be easily disturbed in case of fatigue, sleepiness, or impoverished conditions. When one is sleepy, the second system stops functioning but not the first system.

How do words express our thoughts, feelings, and emotions? Electrical and chemical changes in the brain produce thoughts, feelings, and emotions which in turn cause the activation of the motor nerves. This activated nerve system causes the action of the mouth muscles. Words are produced with the coordination of mouth muscles as they move and as air is exhaled. Physiologically, the voice is controlled by the cerebral cortex and corpus callosum in the brain. When words are heard, the same pattern of stimulation is caused in the corresponding area of the brain. Through this pattern of activation in the brain we can reproduce thoughts, feelings, and emotions similar to those which were created in another's brain. In this way, words or voices are able to convey thoughts, feelings, and emotions.

All words are made of vowels and consonants. However, the main parts of any word are vowels. When you produce vowels you exhale from the abdomen but when you produce consonants, you exhale from the mouth. Consonants are sounds produced merely by mouth movement but vowels are produced by the whole body. Therefore, in any language, vowels are the foundation of words. Roughly speaking, any language consists of five vowels: *AEIOU.* Here, *A* is an *ah* sound, *E* is *eh, I* is *ee, O* is *oh,* and *U* is *ooo.*

In order to produce these sounds, a specific area of the brain must be activated. Specifically, *A* as a sound is the result of the frontal lobe function; the *E* sound is the result of the parietal lobe function; *I* is the result of the central lobe function; *O* is the result of the temporal lobe and cerebellum functions; and finally, *U* is the result of the corpus callosum and brain stem function.

In other words, whenever the sound of *A* is produced, the frontal lobe has been stimulated. Even when the sound of *A* is heard, the frontal lobe is stimulated. Furthermore, each vowel stimulates its corresponding area of the brain which produces particular thoughts, feelings, and emotions.

For example, the frontal lobe reveals the highest function of brain capacities such as abstraction, aspiration, imagination, wonderful feeling, and gratitude. The parietal lobe reveals or is associated with recognition, intellect, and discrimination. The central lobe is associated with sense perception. The temporal lobe and cerebellum are associated with emotion, volition, and action. The corpus callosum, the interbrain, and the brain stem are associated with mechanical, intuitive, and autonomic activities.

The judgment of abstraction, aspiration, imagination, wonderful feeling, and gratitude are improved or stimulated by hearing the *A* sound or voicing the *A* sound. In Sanskrit, *A* is an original life force. In the Shingon sect of Buddhism, Aji (Word) Meditation concentrates on the meaning of *A.* In

English, the article *a* means wonderful and aspiration. The English article *a* must start with wonderfulness; someone finds *a* bread on the table when he is hungry. So he says, "Oh! A bread" instead of saying, "Oh! The bread." Since *the* has the sound of *I*, this corresponds to sense. In other words, *the* bread means that the bread contains a certain smell, color, and shape so that it is distinguished from other breads. Therefore, sensory perception is improved by voicing *I*. The *E* sound relates to recognition, intellect and memory as used in words such as memory, education, knowledge, etc. Therefore, the judgment of intellect, recognition, and memory is improved by the voicing of *E*. The *O* sound relates to emotion, volition, and action as expressed in words such as war, go, do. Therefore, action is strengthened by voicing the *O* sound. Animals snarl before they jump on their prey. The *U* sound relates to intuition and autonomic activities. When we have pain we will say "uuuuu," holding the painful part. The intuitive and autonomic activities are improved by the voicing of *U*.

Summary:

A: Produced with the mouth wide open – when we are surprised or admiring.

E: We produce this sound when we are inquiring.

I: This sound is made when we describe things by using adjectives such as pretty, pity, etc. Japanese adjectives almost always finish with *i*.

O: An action sound. Animals attack their prey with the sound of *o*.

U: This sound is a sound of life. When you have pain you will say *uu*. Japanese verbs almost always finish with 'u.' The regular stem is 'u,' and the regular conversational form is 'masu.'

The Indian and Chinese languages contain many *A* and *U* sounds. Therefore, they are less sensorial and contain less conceptuality – they are more intuitive than the Western languages which contain much *E* sound which makes Westerners more analytical and conceptual. The Japanese language contains many *I* sounds; it is soft, sensitive, delicate. It is very beneficial for Easterners to learn the Western languages and for Westerners to learn the Eastern languages.

April 1972

Cutting Redwoods

Since publishing the decision for cutting selected redwood trees on our property at Mirimichi, I have received several letters from friends and members of the Foundation opposing this act. After receiving these letters, the Board of Directors discussed the matter and consulted with other people. Here is the conclusion of this investigation.

Arguments against cutting the redwood trees or other trees will be considered from two points. One is the standpoint of man, and the other is the standpoint of the tree.

From the standpoint of man: Man cannot live without cutting wood for his needs, just as man cannot live without cutting grains and vegetables for food. However, overcutting of trees will cause the loss of surface soil, the shortage of oxygen, and other factors resulting in environmental destruction. Therefore, we have to find the balancing point between cutting and not cutting. This is exactly what we want to do.

When a redwood forest is logged, a great burst of new trees will sprout up, far more than can be supported to maturity. This has occurred at Mirimichi, where most of the redwoods grow in the eastern and northern parts of the property. They are so dense that even animals can hardly pass through. The percentage of redwood trees is about 10% of the total tree growth in the whole area. We will cut only redwood and fir trees bigger than 20 inches in diameter, which are estimated to be about 3% of all the trees. Therefore, we expect this logging will deteriorate neither the soil nor the environment.

The oldest redwoods growing now are about 60 years old. Therefore, a harvesting was done about 60 years ago. However, about 15 trees are growing from two 20-foot diameter burned redwood stumps. These trees are about 30 years old, so a forest fire burned some of the older trees about 30 years ago. This may happen again in a hot summer, especially because the trees are growing so densely. Selective cutting will help prevent such an accident and the loss of such valuable trees, and will make fire fighting easier in the area.

Also, the cutting of crowded trees will bring much more sunshine to the ground and thus encourage gardening by the people living there. This is in the area near the dwellings. It will also greatly help wintertime living by reducing the dampness and chill resulting from the heavy overgrowth which prevents the sun from filtering below to this overcrowded area.

From the standpoint of the tree: Thinning crowded trees helps the remaining trees grow faster because they will have more water, air, and sunshine. No cutting causes overpopulation so weaker trees will die out. After logging, the forest will be much healthier. This is a known fact in tree botany and forestry. Man is selfish if he considers the ecology for man but not for plants.

Some Americans consider the redwood tree as a sacred tree, and work for its preservation with a religious fervor. This attitude makes sense when a virgin stand of centuries-old trees is threatened, especially in a proposed park area. But to say that redwoods should never be logged seems to me similar to the Indian attitude toward the sacred cow. In Calcutta, if a cow sits on a street, all traffic must be stopped because of the people's belief that cows should not be moved by any means. This is too extreme an attitude, caused by misunderstanding of the sacredness of the cow.

In Japan, rice is considered a sacred grain. Therefore,

every Emperor held a national ceremony when the first crop was harvested each season. However, they were not afraid to cut, cook, and eat it. Rice gains its value when it is eaten. Similarly, a tree gains its value when it is used for man. Otherwise, competition among the trees will kill weaker ones before they are used by man. This is not the right way to handle valuable trees.

Proper Food For Man

A swirl of water begins slowly at its periphery, getting faster and faster as it journeys toward the center. The constantly changing world is very much similar to this swirl of water.

About two hundred years ago, Wall Street in New York was surrounded by pasture land and cows were even driven down Broadway. Now, around the middle of the twentieth century, rays from the sun are blocked by numerous skyscrapers and hardly reach the pavement.

In *The Way Our People Lived* (Washington Square Press), William E. Woodward wrote that there were no American currencies among the New England colonies about 300 years ago. The colonists instead paid their bills with commodities. Today, the American dollar is the monetary standard of our modern twentieth century economy.

Food is one of the last remaining strongholds to change in the world. For a long time grains and vegetables have been the products of the sun, the soil, and much labor. It is a fact that the cultivation of grain was one of the most monumental events in the history of man. For thousands of years grains have been man's fundamental food, the food which has distinguished him from the ape.

The earth, however, shifting on its axis and undergoing great climatic changes, slowly created a new picture. Regions previously suited to the cultivation of grain became better suited to feeding animals. Thus, stock farming and dairy food production got its start. This development was the second great event in human history. Since then, two kinds of men have appeared: one herbivorous, the other carnivorous. These two types were distinct in their physiology as well as mentality, a distinction due primarily to the food of each. Two kinds of mentality were produced, as a matter of course bringing about two distinct civilizations – Eastern and Western.

Thousands of years passed. Then one day a Western man, called a scientist, declared that animal food was the most important food for man (a statement which lacked deep understanding). In Western countries the meat industry became one of the largest, in one country producing over two billion dollars, excluding dairy products, because one half of each person's total food had become meat.

The demand for meat has steadily increased, with farmers raising billions of chickens per year and a tenth that number of cattle. Raising animals has required so much more acreage compared to grain or vegetable farming that pasture land is being exhausted in attempts to meet the demands of increased meat consumption. Many a shrewd, business-minded farmer has adopted animal farming without land. This method is called intensive animal farming and has its roots in England, where the amount of grazing land is in inverse proportion to the heavy demand for meat.

In her informative book *Animal Machines,* Ruth Harrison reveals the mass production techniques of these farmers. She throws light on important problems of today, namely: What is good quality food? Who has the right to treat living creatures solely as 'food-converting machines,' etc.? In modern farming, according to Ms. Harrison, animals are no longer left to graze leisurely on green pastures. The picturesque scene of the grass meadowland has instead become a factory of buildings in which jail-like crates are filled with insecticide-sprayed animals. Feed is automatically dispensed with antibiotics already added. The animals have no real life. They are simply machines that produce animal protein. This is clear evidence why much of today's meat is such poor quality.

Ms. Harrison bluntly poses the question, "How can animals produced under such conditions be safe or acceptable human food?" One might reply, "I don't care how bad it is because I don't eat meat." But let us remember, we are not living in isolation. Our neighbors are all eating meat. The average American consumes an amount of meat equal to one half his total food. It is obvious that if the meat is poor quality, man will suffer physically and mentally. Furthermore, isn't this a clue to the violence, lawlessness, riots, and general decline of health? It is on this last point that Ms. Harrison's findings will interest the non-meat-eating person. She makes three recommendations: (1) Safeguard food from soil to plate by excluding additives, the effects of which are not thoroughly tested and understood; (2) Provide the consumer with information to allow him the option of choosing his food; and (3) Reassess the true quality of food. The first and second measures are matters of legislation and the third is a matter of education. We know from man's history that legislation helps little to provide happiness, since laws give birth to yet more laws. Thus, her three recommendations can be condensed into two questions: (1) What is the proper food for man? and (2) How can people find what good food is and not let their taste deceive them?

Let us discuss the first question. Nutritional theories on the quality of food have been sources of disputes and arguments among many authorities. In *A Doctor Explodes Some Health Food Myths – An Interview With Dr. Frederick Stare, M. D.* (chairman of Harvard's Department of Nutrition), published in the June 1967 *Vogue* magazine, Dr. Stare reported that preservatives tested for toxicity are not used unless safe. He refuted the accusation that commercial preservatives are poisonous, arguing that much of the daily variety of food in this country simply would not exist if not for preservatives. On insecticides, Dr. Stare declared that to his knowledge there existed not "a single documented case of ill health, even a stomachache" caused by insecticide, pesticide, or chemical residue in food.

The *National Health Federation Bulletin,* Vol. 8, September 1967, refuted his remarks saying that former Chief of the Environmental Section of the National Cancer Institute W. C. Heuper, M. D., disagreed, stating that although chemical mixtures used as additives and pesticides were not incorporated in foods, many were not adequately tested for carcinogenic properties. He disclosed that present laws require neither the producer, commercial users, nor the FDA to perform tests that would show any carcinogenic properties before the chemical is accepted. (*Medical World News,* February 10, 1967.)

On the matter of soil, Dr. Stare said also in *Vogue* that if we were to compare three carrots – one grown in organically fertilized soil, one a supermarket carrot grown on a large scale truck farm, and another which could have broken through a crack in a sidewalk – we would find all three to be "nutritional equals." Nutritive value, in his opinion, is not affected by the soil – only the "yield, the amount and size produced."

Again the *NHF Bulletin* criticized these remarks, submitting that a soil expert for the FDA, Dr. Homer Hopkins, indicated in a statement that the defense of such thinking (that the nutritive value of crops is unaffected by soil or fertilizer) is not possible and that his own scientific research revealed the contrary. In fact his report "was so embarassing to the FDA that they refused to release it to the public until the NHF demanded it."

It is apparent that such altercations over the quality of food will never end as long as we use sensorial, sentimental, or scientific analytical reasoning. Food good for one person may not be so for another. Food edible in the summer may be harmful in the winter. Moreover, some people are very healthy eating only raw foods; others eating a similar diet become ill.

Man is a product of the vegetal world; the vegetal world is a product of the soil, climate, and environment. Thus, food grown and eaten in our own area nourishes and sustains us for living happily in that particular climate and environment. A condition for health is a harmonious relationship with one's environment, and this is basically determined by eating the food natural to that environment. Here then is a guide for health, and a macrobiotic principle. It applies to insecticides and additives as well, because these chemicals alter food conditions and change the natural products of the environment. Such alterations deprive us of our capacity to adapt to our particular environment and to be immune from disease.

What Ruth Harrison concludes about the quality of food is similar to the macrobiotic principle. However, the importance of grains as man's principal food is missing. Unable to abandon animal food, she claims the necessity of improving the quality of meat – but not the food of man. In my opinion this is the shortcoming of her work.

As it was said at the beginning, intensive animal farming began because of a shortage of land. This problem can be solved by our adopting a diet including grains as our principal food, and in no other way. This is much easier than making the Sahara desert a fertile land which could provide food for more than the world's present population (see *Sahara Conquest*, Richard Baker, Lutterworth Press, London). For us, intensive animal farming is indeed a 'brave new world' and yet it heralds the coming of man's proper principal food – grain.

The second question is the most difficult problem, even for many who have been macrobiotic for several years. Our senses attract us to food that gratifies short-lived pleasures. We are much like the praying mantis who dies after his first sexual experience. Man does everything to satisfy his sensorial cravings even though the pleasure lasts only a few seconds. Therefore, almost all teaching at this point is futile.

Only as we experience sickness, unhappiness, and enslavement for ourselves do we learn. However, there is one thing we can do, and that is the *wu-wei* of Lao Tsu: teaching without teaching.

Wu-Wei

Wu-wei is one of the most famous ideas of Lao Tsu. It is so famous that almost all the intellectual Chinese and Japanese knew this word. Even in the guest rooms of many Japanese temples and homes hang scrolls of this word, *wu-wei*.

In the second chapter of the *Tao Te Ching* this word appears. *Wu* expresses negation, and *wei* is a verb or noun corresponding with the English word *do* (act, deed). However, 'doing nothing' or 'no deed' do not convey Lao Tsu's idea completely.

Heinrich Wallnofer and Anna von Rottauscher, authors of *Chinese Folk Medicine,* say in their rare book that the clue to the mysticism of Lao Tsu is the word *wu-wei,* 'doing but not doing,' though he does not mean 'doing nothing.' According to his ideas, man should be still and passive before the doings of nature, or *Tao* (the Way); he should perform his small daily tasks and not tackle problems when they have become overwhelmingly huge.

This explanation is neither adequate nor thorough enough. Most Japanese understand *wu-wei* as: You must do as if you are not doing. Teach as if you are not teaching. Teach by your deeds and not with words. Cure the sickness as if you are not curing it. In other words, if you treat a sick man and cure only his sickness, he never learns why he became sick and he will fall ill again. Therefore, your efforts are in vain. However, if instead of treating the sickness you teach him the cause of his sickness and how to cure it by himself, then he will not only be able to cure his present sickness, but will also not become sick again. This is the real cure. In this way you are curing sickness, not just treating it. In short, you are not doing in *so,* but doing in *jitsu. So* stands for appearance and *jitsu* for true nature. (See *Jitsu and So,* pp. 121-128.)

From the point of view of the unique principle, *wu-wei* reveals its deepest meaning. In order to explain this word it is necessary to understand the meaning of one of the Seven Principles of the Order of the Universe: Nothing in this world is eternal in the end. Everything is reversed. Beauty changes to ugliness. Good changes to bad. Non-matter (energy) changes to matter. Ease changes to discomfort and vice versa.

Thus, the wise man of high judgment is free from the desire to live a luxurious life or to be famous or powerful. Such a man, after he accomplishes something, neither praises it, possesses it, nor attaches himself to it. When his accomplishments come apart, he never loses his mind or becomes discouraged.

All accomplishments in this world are eventually futile. The realization that all phenomena of this world are ephemeral and transitory is the essential meaning of *wu-wei.* Histories of great empires such as those of the Roman, Aztec, Mayan, Mongolian, etc., serve merely to explain the ultimate nature of such phenomena.

The bigger the success, the bigger the disappointment or downfall if we don't know the law of change.

The tragedy of John F. Kennedy is a good example.

There are other examples, such as George Eastman, who established the camera empire. In spite of his fame and wealth, he was a very unhappy man and ended his life in suicide. How unfortunate.

Professor Robert Oppenheimer, reputable scholar and creator of the atomic bomb that brought World War II to an end, went through three years of tortuous pain following the detonation; a pain that led to the greatest misery of his life.

Recently Oppenheimer died, leaving his name in the annals of history as builder of an atomic bomb which killed 314,848 noncombatants. He attained honor and distinction and was called the greatest scientist; though he achieved so much, he was not a happy man.

Likewise, the inventor of over twelve hundred useful items, Thomas Edison, believed that his inventions would bring people happiness. His fame and wealth were greater than those of the president of the country. Yet, he was dejected in the later years of his life when he realized his inventions had not helped to make people happy.

Mahatma Gandhi of India devoted his life to liberating the Indians from slavery under the British government. He was very discouraged when he realized the Indians wanted neither independence nor freedom.

Alfred Nobel, Swedish industrialist and founder of the Nobel Prize, is another example. *Science News* described him as probably one of the most unhappy men who ever lived. After amassing a huge fortune from the invention of dynamite and smokeless powder, he became terribly conscience-stricken. Written by hand a year before his death on December 10, 1896, his last will directed that most of his vast fortune be used to institute five magnificent international prizes. The article continued: "He was a quirky, strange and complex man. He was sickly for most of his youth. He never married. He resented his formidable father who was a brilliant, though spasmodic, inventor. He had few close friends, no real home, and once said that his biography should begin 'Alfred Nobel's miserable existence should have been terminated at birth by a humane doctor as he drew his first bawling breath.' " What a miserable, unhappy man.

Be aware, then, for our prosperity, happiness, and health turns inevitably to poverty, unhappiness, and sickness. Let us not cling to this ephemeral world, but instead attach ourselves to the Eternal One, which is the Way, *Tao,* or *wu-wei,* the teaching of Lao Tsu.

Yin and Yang

Whenever a new teller attends me at our bank, she asks me the meaning of the word 'macrobiotic,' which is printed on our deposit slip. I usually explain: " 'Macro' is the opposite of 'micro,' so that it means great or big," because most people know 'micro' as used in microscope, microfilm, and so on. Then I continue, saying, " 'Bio' is the Greek word for life; therefore, 'macrobiotic' means a 'great life'."

In this world you can always find something and its opposite. Any western movie must have bad guys as well as good guys. Good guys only does not make a western movie. The more bad the bad guys, the more good the good guys. In other words, we judge good and bad by comparison. If there is no comparison, there is no good or bad. When we say this food is good, we are comparing it to some other foods which we think not so good. If there is only one food in the market, we don't make the judgment of "good."

Now, we use yin and yang instead of good and bad, so that we don't make sentimental valuations. Yin yang is a concept which divides things in two categories (expansive and contractive) without regard for good or bad. There are cases where yin is good, and vice versa. Yang can also be good or bad. However, beginners tend to think yang is good and yin is bad, and like to eat yang foods only. They have a wrong conception of yin and yang.

In order to clarify yin and yang I will tell you my private

experience. About fifteen years ago my wife was suffering from tuberculosis. Since tuberculosis is a contagious disease, she was hospitalized in a sanatorium 70 miles away from my home. I cooked rice, miso soup, and vegetables for her weekly meals and delivered them to her every Saturday. Saturday and Sunday were my days off work at the Chico San factory; however, on Sunday night I baked bread all night at the factory.

One day a friend of mine gave me two pieces of cooked abalone for my wife. I carried them to the hospital but she didn't want to eat them so I brought them back. On the way home, I started to eat them. When I arrived back home, two pieces of abalone were in my stomach. Then I worked at Chico San all night. In the morning, my stomach was a little uneasy but not painful. I finished my job and went home. I slept in the morning and woke up around noon. I had a little pain in the stomach. I thought it was a gas pain, so I ate a salt plum. As soon as the salt plum reached my stomach, my stomach cramped severely. (This is a yang cramp.) It was so painful that I couldn't lay down on the bed. I fell down from the bed. I climbed up on the bed. I fell down. I climbed up, and fell down. Finally I lost consciousness. A friend of mine stopped over to the house, fortunately, and she found me laying on the floor. She took me to a hospital nearby. A doctor examined me, wondering whether I was a drug addict or not, and injected morphine to stop the pain.

The next morning the stomach pain had gone but I had a new pain over the gall bladder. The doctor said I had a gall bladder stone and needed an operation. I refused the operation. For four days I neither ate nor drank, except for a broth they gave me. On the morning of the fifth day, the breakfast consisted of pancakes with syrup, rice cream topped with sugar, and Ceylon tea. I ate it all and took a hot bath. All the pain had gone. I was released that afternoon. A bill came later, charging $800 including the X-ray fee.

The yin yang balance sheet of my illness will be:

Yang	Yin
2 pieces abalone	1 injection of morphine
1 dry salt plum	4 days broth
70 miles driving	3 pancakes with sugar
8 hours breadbaking	1 bowl rice cream with sugar
hot bath	X-ray
stomach cramp	$800

I do not recommend that you follow my example, but I am merely showing how yin and yang can balance.

One way to learn the yin and yang of foods is to experiment and eat various foods, as Ohsawa did. Another way to learn yin and yang in foods is to observe others whose character and constitution can be related to their favored foods.

After learning yin and yang in foods, you can learn yin and yang in more general subjects. In any case, don't make yin or yang conclusions in a hurry. After you have made them, don't hesitate to change them if you find some factors which contradict the present concept.

The Twelve Unifying Principles of Yin and Yang

1. Yin and yang are the two poles of the infinite pure expansion.
2. Yin and yang are produced infinitely and continuously from the infinite pure expansion itself.
3. Yin is centrifugal; yang is centripetal. Yin, centrifugal, manifests expansion, lightness, cold, dark, etc. Yang, centripetal, manifests constriction, weight, heat, light, etc.
4. Yin attracts yang; yang attracts yin.
5. All phenomena are composed of yin and yang in different proportions.

6. All phenomena are constantly changing their yin and yang components. Everything is restless.

7. There is nothing completely yin or completely yang. All is relative.

8. There is nothing neuter. There is always yin or yang in excess.

9. Affinity or force of attraction between things is proportional to the difference of yin and yang in them.

10. Yin repels yin; yang repels yang. The greater the difference, the weaker the repulsion.

11. Yin eventually becomes yang and yang eventually becomes yin.

12. Everything is yang at its center and yin at its periphery (surface).

Jitsu and So

The Order of the Universe is expressed in seven laws, one of which states: *That Which Has a Front Has a Back.* What is the relation between this law of universal logic and the two antagonistic categories, yin and yang?

To begin with, this law tells us that if the face (front) is yang, the back is yin. In other words, front and back are not only different from each other but are opposite or antagonistic.

In the Far East, front and back are known by two words: *jitsu* and *so*. *Jitsu* (back) means inner nature or true nature (intrinsic). *So* (front) means outward or apparent nature (extrinsic).

Jitsu and *So* of the Heart

There are four chambers in the heart. What is the yin yang order of these four chambers – right and left auricle, right and left ventricle?

Since the left ventricle forces the blood through the whole body, this must be the most yang. In reality, the muscular wall of the left ventricle is the thickest. The most yin chamber must be the right auricle, because it is opposite in position to the left ventricle. The muscular wall of this chamber is the most thin. Likewise, the right ventricle is more yang than the left auricle because the right ventricle forces the blood longer distances than the left auricle does. Therefore, the order is as follows:

Most Yin – right auricle
Yin – left auricle
Yang – right ventricle
Most Yang – left ventricle

Examine this order carefully. You will notice two things:

(1) The order of the blood flow is yin-yang-yin-yang because it starts at the right auricle (yin) and flows to the right
ventricle (yang) to the left auricle (yin) and finally to the left
ventricle (yang).

(2) As a whole, the left side is more yang than the right
side. This is certain because blood containing oxygen (yin)
comes in the left side of the heart and blood containing carbon dioxide (yang) comes in from the right side of the heart.

From the standpoint of Oriental philosophy the above is
contradictory, because it is said that the right is yang and left
is yin. This is the reason the heart (yang) is located on the
left side of the body (yin). This can be explained as follows:
The right side of the heart is more yin in its true nature than
the left side; however, the right side contains yang blood.
Therefore, in the end, the apparent nature of the right side
becomes yang. In other words, the yin yang order of the heart
is inverted when we consider it with or without blood. We
always observe the heart with blood. This is what is apparent,
or *so*.

	Jitsu (without blood)	So (with blood)
Left side of heart	Yang	Yin
Right side of heart	Yin	Yang

Jitsu and *so* of the hydrogen atom

Is the hydrogen atom yin or yang?

The atomic transmutation theory tells us that all elements are transmuted from hydrogen through a spiralling journey beginning at the periphery and moving toward the center – in other words, a centripetal spiral. That is to say, everything that begins yin ends yang in this spiralling journey. From this point of view, hydrogen must be the most yin element. However, George Ohsawa defined hydrogen as a yang element according to its spectroscopic analysis. How can we solve this contradiction?

The beginning of the centripetal spiralling orbit corresponds to that which is called an electron in modern physics. The various points of this orbit could be considered as the various elementary particles. The energy which is called the electron arrives at its terminus and changes to a proton (yang). Since this proton is yang it attracts electrons to form hydrogen. Because the difference of yin and yang between the electron and proton is great, their combination is strong and stable, thus producing the yang element, hydrogen. However, yang attracts yin and as soon as they form hydrogen it attracts space (yin) and attains a gaseous state (yin). Therefore, we can only observe the gaseous state of hydrogen which is in the yin state. Being observable, it is *so*.

However, the *jitsu* (true nature, or back, of hydrogen) is yang.

Jitsu and *so* of summer

The summer is hot. Its *jitsu* is yang. Plants, vegetables, and trees grow and provide shade. Its *so* is yin.

Jitsu and *so* of man and animal

Man stands upright. His *so* is yin. What is his *jitsu*?
The animal crawls. His *so* is yang. What is its *jitsu*?

Jitsu and *so* of men

A rich man is rich as his *so*; therefore, his *jitsu* must be poor. Since he is poor, he saves and clings to everything to be rich. A poor man is poor in his *so*; therefore, his *jitsu* must be rich. Since he is rich in *jitsu*, he doesn't save or cling to anything but instead gives away everything freely and becomes poor.

The happy man is an unhappy man in reality because his *so* (happiness) must change to unhappiness. If you want to be happy all the time, your *so* and *jitsu* must be happy. To be happy in *jitsu* you must make your *so* unhappy. In other words, always try to solve the most difficult problems.

The unhappy man is happy in reality because his *so* (unhappiness) must change to happiness. There is only one requirement for this. It is patience. Psychological patience is born of physiological patience. Give the body (it is animal) the longest and hardest task – to build itself. Specifically, eat from the vegetable world: grains and vegetables. Let the body change itself into man (the animal world). This process requires more patience from us than if we were to just eat animal products such as meat, fish, and dairy products. For the person who eats meat, there is no substantial change required; therefore, there will be no patience developed.

If you have patience, there is no unhappiness in this world because all unhappiness inevitably changes to happiness sooner or later. There are only difficulties which are like a mathematical exercise. The difficult problems give us more joy when we solve them.

Man, animal, plants, air, water, light, etc., are all different in their *so* but their *jitsu* is the same. We call it Oneness or Infinity.

Jitsu and *so* in the I Ching

A hexagram of the I Ching shows *jitsu* and *so*. The upper

part of the hexagram is *so* and the lower part of the hexagram is *jitsu*. For example, Hexagram No. 11, 'Tai – Peace'

☷ *So* (front)

☰ *Jitsu* (back)

(above – the receptive, earth;
below – the creative, heaven)
reveals that the front (*so*) is yin
and the back (*jitsu*) is yang.
That is why in this hexagram everything is successful, because *jitsu* is yang (aggressive) and *so* is yin (passive). Yin
appears in the yin position (upper part). Yang appears in the
yang position (lower part). Therefore, this hexagram shows
everything is in good order.

If this hexagram represented a married couple, the lower
part (yang) would represent the husband and the upper part
(yin) the wife. When the husband is very yang, works hard,
is brave and strong, and his wife is yin – gentle, patient, and
delicate – then the family is in good order, is happy and
healthy. Such a family can be described as a tree with strong
roots. The root is the yang back which nurtures the beautiful
flower, the yin front. Without strong roots, a tree cannot grow
and blossom – and yet we do not see the roots. Thus, the root
is the back of the tree. The flower is beautiful and attractive.
It is the first thing we notice about a tree; therefore, it is the
front. However, if the flower were dark, coarse, and tough
like a root we would never appreciate it. By the same token, if
a root were delicate and gentle as a flower, the tree would
soon die.

Thus, if the back is yang and the front is yin, we have good
order. This hexagram has been considered to be the most
fortunate of all the sixty-four hexagrams in China and Japan.

Jitsu and *so* of our constitution

We grow three billion times in our mother's womb, during
which time we feed solely on our mother's blood. After birth
we grow only twenty times. Thus our constitution is pre-
dominately formed during the fetal period and is called the
inherited constitution. It is like the root of the tree. This con-

stitution is considered basic, or the 'back' constitution.

If this basic constitution is yang, we attract yin after our birth and acquire a yin constitution on the surface or in appearance. This is the 'front' of one's constitution. To illustrate: a girl is more yang than a boy by birth; therefore she is attracted to more yin food after birth and she becomes feminine while maturing. However, she has a basically yang 'back' and therefore is naturally domestic, stable, patient, sentimental, and sensorial. She is acquiring her femininity and delicacy, which is her 'front' later. Thus, physiologically, woman's 'front' is yin and 'back' is yang.

A boy is opposite. He is more yin than a girl by birth and is therefore attracted to more yang food and acquires yang manliness in maturity. Thus, psychologically, man's 'front' is yang and his 'back' is yin physiologically.

Everything changes. This is the law of nature. However, some things change quickly, others change more slowly; in ten days our red blood cells change, but our body cells change every seven years. We can consider that blood is the 'front' factor of the physical constitution, whereas all body cells are the 'back' factor of the physical constitution.

How can we change our blood? Change what you eat and the blood changes. This changes the symptoms of the illness. This change is the 'front' of sickness. The real cure comes after all cells change. This is the 'back'.

How do we change yin cells to yang cells? Eating yang foods is not enough, because just changing the quality of our blood results in a condition where the 'front' is yang and the 'back' is yin.

Here is the reason that many in macrobiotics reveal rigidity, arrogance, false confidence, laziness, disorderliness, joylessness, lack of gratitude, and exclusiveness in spite of their sickness disappearing. Their body cells which they had produced previous to the macrobiotic diet, many years ago, had not become yang. To me, this appears to be the shortcoming or disadvantage of the diet. In other words, this is the result of a disorder between 'front' and 'back'. We must make the 'back' yang, not the 'front'. One should be gentle, smiling, cheerful, and flexible on the 'front' – but strong, steady, patient, and brave at the 'back'. This is not an easy job. But, without this order we will never be happy.

Of course, our cells change gradually. It is a slow process. Yet, how can we make yang cells quickly?

(1) Yangize without food. Yangize by doing some activity; i. e., hard physical work, doing things for others, etc. Keep yourself busy.

(2) Surround the body by yin or place yourself in yin conditions. Eat little. Wear little. Live in a cold climate. Seek difficulties if you don't have any. Leap into new environments or situations which provide you with a big challenge. Should you have difficulties now, consider yourself a happy man who has been given the best conditions to be happy.

(3) Open your eyes, look closely, see the sky, flowers, birds, fish, animals, trees, and grass. Express these in any form, such as a song, a poem, a picture, a drawing, music, writing – and do it without any sentiment or sensory judgment. This will lead you to detachment of ego. (In Japan such an expression was called haiku.) Most art is expression of the sensorial or sentimental level of judgment.

Jitsu and *so* of macrobiotics

The aim of macrobiotic life is happiness. Two types of people observe macrobiotics, just as there are two kinds of happiness one may aim for. These are the *so* and *jitsu*, both aiming at a happy life. *So* happiness is symptomatic; *jitsu* happiness is true and everlasting. Most people take the symptomatic approach – the removal of pain or sickness, getting rid of symptoms. When the pain stops, they leave macrobiotics. This is the same idea as a drug store, using macrobiotics like they would use drugs. Such people cannot continue macrobiotics.

One of my students asked why George Ohsawa continued

macrobiotics for fifty years. I told him that Mr. Ohsawa had a very bad sickness and cured himself with macrobiotics. He was so grateful to the diet and the principle that he decided he would help other people by teaching this principle. However, without gratitude, regardless of what you accomplish, you will never be happy. True happiness is basically gratitude. For this we need good health, for it is hard to feel gratitude when you are sick. All of us need to learn how to become grateful.

In Japan, many thousands of people have been cured by macrobiotics. There are more than six hundred different books written and published by Mr. Ohsawa, but none of these can be found in used book stores. People are keeping them. However, there are only a few active in macrobiotics; most are only using it for a symptomatic cure.

How does one acquire gratitude? (1) Education in childhood. Parents teaching by example. (2) Difficulties. In trying to overcome and accept responsibility for all his difficulties, one learns gratitude.

Jitsu and *so* of difficulties and happiness

We must not blame viruses, microbes, lack of money, or society for our unhappiness. Of difficulties, there are two kinds. *Jitsu* (true) difficulties are imposed by yourself, and *so* difficulties are imposed from the outside (by others). When you overcome *so* difficulties you get *so* happiness. When you overcome *jitsu* difficulties you get *jitsu* happiness. *So* happiness is never made by us, so there is no true gratitude. However, *jitsu* happiness produces true gratitude. When you overcome *so* difficulties, happiness is *so* or symptomatic happiness. A good example is science and medicine offering *so* cures, and thus offering only *so* happiness. *So* happiness using pills or surgical techniques is happiness obtained through others.

We must attain *jitsu* happiness, not *so*. This is the genuine, true, and everlasting happiness.

How Did Religion Start?

A friend and I were guests on a morning television show. When we were there, the host was answering questions about state tax problems. We were told that our show would also be like that. Many questions would be asked through telephone calls. I was not nervous but expected many challenges.

After a few questions, the host asked us what benefits we get from the macrobiotic diet. This question puzzled me because I have been on this diet for so long, I have almost forgotten what I am getting from the macrobiotic diet.

Macrobiotic eating is like air, light, and water without which we cannot live. Yet it is difficult to say what we get from air, light, and water. It seems a silly question to ask someone who is enjoying having it so much. No reply can adequately answer this question. Therefore, whatever I answer will probably not be accurate. For the public, however, such questions and answers are most important to know because the majority of people will be attracted to macrobiotics by what they will get from it. In modern society, people are concerned about what they receive rather than what they give. They try to receive as much as possible, giving as little as possible.

In order to attract the public, therefore, one must promise what they will get for their efforts. In politics, candidates promise prosperity to the voters. In education, schools promise students good income. In medicine, doctors promise cures for patients. And in religion, priests promise believers a happy life, whatever that may mean. In other words, religions promise people tangible results through practice of that religion.

I will examine how religion starts from this point.

In ancient China, the art of rejuvenation developed. This art of rejuvenation was called *sendo* – the way of *sennin*. The mountain sages who practiced it were the *sennin* (mountain men). *Sen* is made of two ideograms: 山, mountain, and 人, man. Therefore, 仙 (*sen*) means mountain man which is opposed to 俗. Here, 谷 is valley and 人 is man. Therefore, 俗 (*zoku*) means valley man.

Sen and *zoku* will be clearly understood using yin yang philosophy. From the standpoint of yin and yang, the valley is a closed, limited world. Therefore, valley man means an unfree, attached man who has low judgment. Fear, anxiety, quarrels, and eventually sickness and unhappiness are the result. On the other hand, the mountain is open and has unlimited view. Mountain man, then, means a free man who has high judgment that can see through time and space. He knows the cause of all results. He has no anxiety, fear, violence, sickness, or unhappiness.

Sendo consists of five arts. The first one was *do-in* – physical exercises which make our body healthy and flexible. The second art was diet. The Chinese recommended moderate amounts of necessary foods, locally grown – avoiding foods which are based on sensorial taste, desire, and stimulation. The third art was breathing. It was understood that breathing gives us life. Breathing was therefore an important art in creating rejuvenation of the body.

All these three are physical arts.

The fourth one was meditation on the inner body. The Chinese believed that our body, organ, and muscle functions are controlled by 36,000 gods. Palaces where each god lives are called *kyu* – points of acupuncture. When the gods are in these palaces, we are healthy. Sickness comes when the gods leave these palaces. Any medicine or exercise is of no use if it cannot keep these gods in the palaces. In order to keep the gods there, the Chinese recommended understanding the action, mechanism, and function of each point. Chinese medicine and its meridian system developed from this meditation.

The fifth art is understanding or having an awareness of a principal god, the utmost god which produces and controls these 36,000 gods in our body. This god controls not only our body but also the principal law or order of all phenomena. Therefore, awareness or clear understanding in daily life (not conceptual understanding) of life's order is the last aim of *sendo*: free man.

Lao Tsu named this one god *tao*: the order or law of all phenomena. It is invisible; therefore, it is *mu* (no matter, invisible). It manifests itself, however, in all phenomena; therefore, it is *yu* (visible). Life and matter are manifestations of *tao*. Sickness or accident are results of *tao*. So Tsu developed Lao Tsu's philosophy. "All phenomena are relative and changing. There is nothing absolute and static. Beauty and ugliness, good and evil, right and wrong, large and small, long and short are all antagonistic and transmuting phenomena. The law, principle, or order of antagonism, change, and transmutation is *tao*."

Once one understands that his body or mind is a manifestation of this *tao*, then he can understand that he is *tao*. This is the unification of man and *tao*. This is a free man who does not die. He does not suffer from fire, water, or wind. He can see beyond space and time. He can fly and change himself. This is the ultimate aim of *sendo*.

Eventually, the meaning of free man was misunderstood by the valley man who tried to realize these miraculous powers in the limited physical world instead of clearly understanding the meaning of *tao* – order of yin yang. Such misunderstandings were broadened by pseudo-healers, magicians, or leaders who promised the miraculous power of *tao* simply by paying money. This is the origin of the *Tao* religion. The *Tao* religion promises extrasensory perception, telepathic powers, the ability to see past and future, the power of reading minds, the ability to be in two places at one time, being able to change oneself into other forms, to levitate and fly, and to immobilize another person. The Monkey King began his career by learning these powers and finished by becoming a Buddhist. These powers are infinitely small powers of *tao*. People who believe only what they see will be guided or led by these promises. As a result, the *Tao* religion developed and real *tao* was left behind.

The first four arts are a means of realizing supreme judgment – awareness of *tao* – in daily life. This takes real patience and tedious endurance to practice. So the *Tao* religion degenerated by promising magical powers to get people to practice. Human desire and greediness changed the original teaching. Physics and metaphysics became confused. Most organized religions have followed similar downward paths.

Macrobiotics may become a religion if we make a sensorial magical promise. Our host was trying to be helpful during our television appearance. At the time of a station break he said, "Gentlemen, don't be so guarded. Remember, you are trying to sell macrobiotics." He wanted us to promise fantastic results if people would eat brown rice.

When we emphasize miraculous cures of cancer or other sicknesses through macrobiotics, we are forgetting that it is not a miracle at all because the macrobiotic diet is a manifestation of light, water, air – the whole universe or oneness, which is the Creator. By the hand of the Creator, there are no miracles. When we show miraculous abilities resulting from the macrobiotic diet, we are forgetting that we are the creator of life which is the biggest miracle in the universe.

There are other forms of 'sales tricks' in the macrobiotic

movement; that is to say, the concept of *dream*. Ohsawa defined happiness as follows: "Happiness is the infinite realization of all your dreams." Then someone promises this realization if macrobiotics is observed. Many young students carry their life with a big dream in order to be happy. Unfortunately, this promise sometimes makes their daily life miserable, unhappy, and unpleasant because of their having too big a dream.

Don't eat macrobiotically to accomplish some big dream. Don't guide your life by some future goal. Your dreams should be realized in the present, every day. Don't mix up future plans, which are based on a realization of everyday dreams, with a big future dream which has no basis in an everyday plan.

Create Your Own Temple

When I guided Mr. Ohsawa in a town on the East Coast about 15 years ago, he said, "There are so many churches." I visited Japan with 20 macrobiotic Americans this summer. I was amazed and said, "There are so many temples."

Christian churches represent Western mentality, way of life, and environment. Buddhist temples represent Oriental mentality, way of life, and environment. Although there are many differences between churches and temples in construction, architecture, arts, and rituals, I saw many similarities. The biggest similarity is that they are mostly dead. Most of the temples we visited are dead. They are the shell of a cast-out spirit. They are art museums or showplaces where paradise is supposedly exhibited.

Buddha taught a way of life without temples and without priests. Now Buddhism has thousands of temples and priests in Japan alone. Originally, temples were learning places to live and study with a master. Later, temples became schools where one can learn Buddhist chanting and rituals so that he can manage a temple belonging to his sect. Once he manages a temple, his income is secured by the clients of that temple. The more famous the temple, the more clients and income it has. If a priest has talent he can increase his following. The talent he needs is not high understanding of Buddhism or high spirit of salvation but that of how to attract people and how to manage the various rituals, income, and expenditures of temples. Being a priest is being a businessman. Their biggest business is to assure the dead a paradise instead of hell. Everyone dies and does not want to go to hell. So 99.99% of Japanese if not 100% are taken care of by a priest after death. Not only funeral services but early services after death are performed by priests for donations.

The original Buddha's teaching was not like this. He taught we must observe the middle path – without extreme yin and yang in thinking, actions, speech, and eating; that is to say, the Noble Eightfold Path. The real Buddhism is in our mind and heart by which we think and act. Without right thinking and action, we never reach a happy life or death.

Why were so many temples built? Temples were originally built to study Buddhism. To study Buddhism is to overcome insecurity or fear. We have fears because our life is uncertain, tomorrow is unknown. We may have an accident tomorrow, we may lose a job, fortune, wife, or children at any time. I am afraid of another because I do not know how he thinks about me.

In Japanese Buddhism, there are two types of schools to overcome this fear. One type is relying on self-discipline and the other is relying with complete faith on the salvation of Amidha Nyorai which is the same as Christ in Christianity. Schools of self-discipline are for the more intellectual because their teachings are logical, sophisticated, and philosophical. The other school is for the uneducated and it teaches oneness or security through religious self-repentance without any logical explanation. For modern people, the latter seems superstitious. However, it has acquired more followers than the other. It has accumulated more power and wealth, not through the higher spirit of preachers or doctrines but through the almost blind faith of massive numbers of followers. One person advised a follower that his donation to the temple is useless because the priest may use his money wrongly or selfishly. The follower replied, "I am donating because I am happy and my happiness is caused by Buddha's salvation. I like to keep the temple where Buddha stays. I don't care whether the priest uses my money selfishly or not."

Their faith in the salvation of Amidha Nyorai is strong as a rock. Therefore, they have no fear and they are happy. On the other hand, other schools which try to reach the state of no fear through self-discipline such as *zazen*, meditation, chanting, and discussion of doctrines seem to me less successful. Why? These teachings are logical, rational, and intellectual. Logic, rationality, and intellect lead us to an analytical attitude which divides everything – yin and yang, you and I, God and man, etc. The intellectual mind understands oneness but he is not oneness or happiness. Understanding is different from being. Religion is to become a happy being which is different from the understanding of happiness. Modern people, especially Westerners, need understanding to acquire faith. Then how to unite the being with intellectual understanding? How can the ego unite with the egoless God, Buddha, or Nature?

One who reaches faith in Buddha or the Order of the Universe without any intellectual thinking is a lucky one. However, most of our modern people have too much knowledge and education to do this. We need some other approach. Religious practice such as *zazen*, meditation, or chanting is not essential, from my experience. The essential thing is our thinking, behavior, and action which reveal the innermost light of our Buddha nature. In other words, we must think, behave, and act upon the light or wisdom of Buddha nature, and we all have this nature. It is just buried in the subconscious mind due to our education and customary living. What does it mean to reveal the light of Buddha nature?

Just eating good foods is not enough to be a happy person. How we pay the cost of foods, for example, is important. If we pay by money, we are not revealing the light of Buddha nature because we cannot pay the cost of foods just by money.

The value of foods is priceless – it is a gift from heaven and earth. It was produced by sunshine, water, soil, bacteria, and sweat. If our payment in money doesn't contain sweat, we are cheating. It becomes our debt. We are living in debt from birth to death. We have to pay this debt as soon as possible, otherwise we are not free. However, we never clear up our debt because it is infinite. Therefore we have to live in infinite appreciation. This infinite appreciation is the light of Buddha nature, the light of Bliss.

The revealing of this light is creating a temple. We have to build our own temple where the eternal light of Bliss shines.

The Art of Cooking

Cooking is an art that creates joy, pleasure, delicious taste, beauty, and friendship as well as health and happiness. If cooking is not an art, then what is art? For cooking to be an art, the cuisine must be delicious, well harmonized, and beautifully decorated. To make her cooking an art, a woman must develop her aesthetic sense so that it will be revealed not only in her cooked food but also in her kitchen, at the dinner table, and even in the garbage can. Such an aesthetic sense is especially required in the Japanese tea ceremony, where the eye must be sensitive enough to see the sights that mark the way to follow. Such signs may be a cleaned footpath, a clean wet footstone washed by water, or a broken branch. Such signs will lead you to the teahouse, but if your aesthetic sense is not sharp, you may get lost.

In the teahouse, you see a scroll hanging on the *tokonoma* (a special wall of the guest room used for the scroll) and flowers arranged in front of it. These are the host's special decorations which match the season and feeling of the occasion. In the center of the room there is a fireplace carved into the floor. Black charcoals burn red and their white ashes partly cover them. The room is so quiet that you can hear outside breezes. Such a setting is part of the preliminary preparation and is essential to the art of the tea ceremony.

Cooking and serving a dinner must be performed with the same aesthetic sense. The admiration and disciplined effort to develop such a sense is called *do* as in *judo, kyudo* (the art of archery), *kado* (flower arrangement), *shodo* (brush painting), *kendo* (fencing or swordsmanship), *aikido,* and *ido* (the art of medicine). Such aesthetic education in the mastering of the arts is best described and illustrated in the August 1960 issue of *House Beautiful* magazine:

> Nothing in our Western world can compare with the role that aesthetics has played in Japanese life for 1,200 years. The Japanese prized sensitivity to beauty since the 8th century. An important word in their vocabulary of aesthetics is 'aware,' and generally means sensitivity to things or subtlety of discrimination. One writer called it the "ah-ness" of things. The Japanese have not distinguished between the beautiful and practical, with the result that their most commonplace objects are worth paying serious attention to as aesthetic achievement. Every necessity is considered as a chance to have beauty. They have developed a condition and an attitude to beauty which has made of it something to consume and experience every hour of every day. . . .
>
> Their non-separation of the beautiful from the practical seemed to us completely ideal. Their subtlety of discrimination of beauty intrigued us particularly. Four of their words for beauty we have made our own (*shibui, jimi, iki, and hade*), and they have been valuable in helping us think more precisely about beauty and its many forces.
>
> One of these words, *shibui,* (an adjective) has the highest connotations, and we devote 20 pages in this issue to its meaning. (A quick translation of *shibui* is 'a severe exquisiteness.')

The four Japanese words for beauty can be explained by the concept of yin and yang. *Hade* is brightly colored, bold patterned, exuberant in overall effect, is yang, and is considered an immature, youthful aesthetic sense. *Jimi,* the opposite of *hade,* is sober and sedate in color; proper, correct, and therefore dull. There is no 'showing off,' no character. This can be considered yin. There is *iki*, between the above two types of beauty. *Iki* is the Japanese equivalent of the French word *chic:* smart, stylish, a la mode, clever, and sophisticated. *Iki* is more yin than *hade*, but more yang than *jimi*.

Shibui is the beauty of no comparisons. It is absolute, beyond yin and yang. According to *House Beautiful:*

> It is unobtrusive and unostentatious, intrinsically good. Most Japanese strive to achieve *shibui* in their dress and other possessions. Probably 60% achieve only *jimi*. *Shibui* takes more depth of understanding than *jimi*. They get the words but not the tune, and achieve only proper correctness. *Shibui* is the essence of Japanese culture and is considered the ultimate in taste – for all but the very young. The characteristics of *shibui* are described as follows:
>
> 1. Simple, with an economy of line and effort. Nothing complicated could be *shibui*.
> 2. Must have depths worth studying, after first being noticed.
> 3. Must be a fitting exploitation of the nature of the material and the method.
> 4. Should not be shiny or new looking, though small touches of sparkle can be used.
> 5. It is aimed to produce tranquility.
> 6. A feeling of modesty or humility is necessary in striving for *shibui*.

Such beauty is the ultimate in all arts in Japan. *Kado* or *sado* (tea ceremony) are examples of the discipline or self-education leading to the realization of such beauty in everyday life. *Judo, aikido, kendo, and kyudo* are the disciplines which strive to achieve modesty and humility instead of force or power in our daily life. *Shodo* or *edo* are disciplines to realize such beauty in writing or painting. *Haikudo* ('poem-writing art') is a discipline to realize such beauty in poetry. The mastery of the art of cooking is called *ryorido* in Japanese. *Ryorido* is a discipline aimed at achieving beauty, taste, and humility in cooking and diet. The master of this art, therefore, must attain the beauty, taste, modesty, and humility of *shibui*. *Do* is the Japanese equivalent of the Chinese *tao*. The macrobiotic diet and cooking is called *shokuyodo*, the way of eating and cooking to reach the highest health and happiness.

Two Kinds of Memories

There are two kinds of memories: the memories of joy and the memories of sadness. George Ohsawa often said that good memory is the foundation of our happiness. However, if we live with sad memories, we are sad. Therefore, he meant that a good memory must be a joyous one and not a sad one. How can we live with a joyous memory all the time when we have an unpleasant memory too?

To solve this, some modern psychotherapists emphasize the concept of 'here and now.' Since unhappy people are living with memories of sadness, resentment, and discontent, they are happier when they can forget those memories. The concept of 'here and now' is a help for them. However, if we emphasize 'here and now' indiscriminately, we may end up with persons who have no past (the foundation of the present). The concept of 'here and now' may solve many problems that modern people suffer from; at the same time, it may create a person who forgets benefits received in the past. This creates an ungrateful person and in turn his happiness is not real. In other words, 'here and now' must be full of memories of joy and gratitude of the past.

Recently, I met a girl I have known for quite a long time. She had been a sad and introverted person. But she was very joyous and outgoing this time. She said this change has been brought about not by macrobiotics but by a mental training she had recently undertaken. The mental training wiped out her conceptual yin and yang thinking and made her attitude less rigid. So far everything was fine and beautiful. Her mental training created a great change in her. I admitted this and I admire the training she received. When we talked she said, "I think your macrobiotic publications are all a waste of time and effort. They don't bring any good. Why do you keep publishing?"

I was shocked. I felt deeply sorry she saw things in that way. I was sorry because she felt she had not benefited from macrobiotics. I admit that my writing or lectures are not strong enough to change the mental attitude of people who suffer from sad memories. This is not a fault of macrobiotics but of me; many people have benefited from the diet and way of life taught by macrobiotics. She must have benefited too. She has forgotten the past when she came to me asking help at first. At that time she was so unhappy and sick. Without macrobiotics she would not have avoided serious sickness for the past several years. Without macrobiotics, she would have been more miserable. She had been picking up sad memories. Therefore, the concept 'here and now' worked nicely. However, this created an ungrateful person too. If this is the case, 'here and now' is not a final solution to our mental attitude. We have to develop a concept of life that is deeper and higher: that is to say, the 'supreme judgment' of Ohsawa.

This supreme judgment, which is unforgettable gratitude, is too difficult for many sick Americans. Their lives have been full of continual complaints and much sadness. Therefore, 'here and now' is one solution for them: Never mind the past, we live in the 'here and now.' Actually, this attitude is but the first step toward the supreme judgment or eternal happiness which we are all aiming at. As long as we stay at 'here and now' only, our happiness does not last long. It will fade away sooner or later. In order to develop our mental attitude from 'here and now' to everlasting happiness, we have to learn how to memorize and appreciate the past. A girl told me once that she could not appreciate everything because her past was unpleasant. How can we live in appreciation even though we are full of sadness from the past?

To solve this question, we must think about the mechanism of memory. It is our consciousness which picks memories out of the storehouse of joyous or sad memories. Without the function of consciousness, memory is not 'here and now.' When I was a student I went mountain climbing and fell from a rock about 30 feet. Within a second, I recalled thousands of events in my past. This is the function of consciousness. That time my consciousness picked up memories without discrimination. However, consciousness usually picks them with a choice – either joyous ones or sad ones. If consciousness would always pick up the joyous memories, we would be happy. How can this be possible?

First, we have to make our blood yang or alkaline so that the sad memories, which are yin, will be neutralized and will not reach consciousness. If our blood is acid or yin, it will expel yin memories, bringing them to consciousness. Second, we have to exercise an attitude which picks only joyous memories with appreciation. This is prayer. Third, we have to elevate our consciousness so that it can transmute sad memories to joyous ones.

George Ohsawa had much suffering and unhappiness and yet he lived with the memories of joyfulness. He was a happy and free man. Our consciousness and diet can do this. He proved it. Let us cultivate such consciousness.

I have recently received a letter from a mother of two girls whom I don't remember. (What a bad memory I have.) She wrote in her letter, "I don't know if you remember, but about 2 years ago our oldest daughter fell and was unconscious when we found her. We did not know what had happened to her and did not know what to do. It was through your and Cornellia's help that we were reassured and had the confidence to do as you instructed. My husband and I will never forget you."

What happy people they are. They are happy because they remember the accident, the help, and the recovery. They could be sad by just memorizing the accident. They could be 'happy' by forgetting all of the incident. It is the choice of our memory whether we are happy or not. This choice depends on our physical condition and consciousness (judgment). By our judgment, memory of the past becomes present, here and now. Let us live here and now with a deep grateful memory.

Giving My Books a Home

We live in air, sunshine, on soil, and surrounded by wood, grass, buildings, noise, etc. We are also surrounded by unseen radiations and energies. These are all material surroundings. However, there is also another kind: we live in a spiritual environment.

To understand this I will tell you an experience I had recently. When I was living in San Francisco I could read and write well. Then we moved to Vega, in the foothills of the Sierra Nevada mountains. Here the air and water are very clean. Our nearest neighbor was miles away. In this fresh and quiet environment I could not read or write. I thought the reason was that I was too busy managing two organizations – the farm and the publishing house in Oroville.

Every morning I would drive the 45 minutes to the Foundation, work all day, drive home to the farm, then do garden work or house and car repair. It was a busy routine, but always before I found time for reading and writing. At the farm I couldn't.

After selling the Vega farm, we moved to Oroville. My life became much easier. I had more time to relax. Still, I could not read or write. I didn't understand why. I thought perhaps I had become too yang – older.

In the new home I recently made shelves for my many books accumulated over the years. I arranged them in an orderly way and got rid of the books I didn't want. As soon as

I put my books in order I started to read and write again. I remembered that at Vega when my room was well organized I could read and write. However, because many students lived in the house my books were spread all around and I never had my own study room.

Books are printed thoughts and ideas of the author. When we read a book we make contact with the author. The thoughts and ideas on the pages are not confined there; they drift up and surround us. This creates a spiritual environment. Therefore, it is important for a happy life that we are surrounded by spiritually guiding books. If you are surrounded by angry, mean, and resentful books, you become an angry, mean, and resentful person. If you are surrounded by healthy and joyful books, you become such a person.

George Ohsawa sent me many books from Japan. He also gave me many books when he stayed in my apartment in New York. Many other friends have given me books. All these have special meaning for me. When I see them I contact not only the author, but also the person who gave me the book. When I read my copy of the *Tao Te Ching*, I live with Lao Tsu, and at the same time I recall the friend who gave me the book. This is my spiritual environment which is full of appreciation, joy, and happiness.

Great Paradoxes in Man

> Words that are strictly true
> seem to be paradoxical.
> *The Tao Te Ching*

Eric Fromm refers to the logic of Lao Tsu and Buddha as paradoxical logic because it assumes that A and non-A do not exclude each other as predicates of X. He states, "Paradoxical logic was predominant in Chinese and Indian thinking, in the philosophy of Heraclitus, and then again under the name of dialectics it became the philosophy of Hegel, and of Marx."

Here are some examples from the New Testament:

> He that findeth his life shall lose it; and he that loseth his life for my sake shall find it. (Matthew X:39)

> For whosoever hath, to him shall be given, and he shall have more abundance; but whosoever hath not, from him shall be taken away even that which he hath. (Matthew XIII:12)

We find similar sayings in Zen:

> Master Basho said to the monks, "If you have a stick, I will give you one; if you don't have a stick, I will take it away from you." (44th case of the Mumon-kan.)

In order to understand these sayings, one must understand the constitution of life. Life has two aspects: one is relative life which is tangible, ephemeral, egoistic, pain/pleasure, stress/relaxed. The other is infinite, absolute, universal, intangible, eternal, One. In Matthew X:39, the reference is to the eternal life. Matthew XIII:12 means that whoever understands eternal life will enjoy his relative life. But he who does not understand eternal life will live his relative life in sickness and unhappiness. One who sees life as only relative and individual cannot cure sickness or attain true happiness. Ohsawa taught yin and yang so that one can realize a big life ('macrobiotics'), like that which is taught in the Bible, Zen, and in Buddhism.

I recently found another great paradox in life: that of conscious and subconscious. I see, smell, and hear things. These are all results of my conscious mind at work. Their experiences will be stored in my subconscious mind. The functions of the conscious and subconscious are in great paradox.

The consciousness is constantly receiving ever-changing impulses. The impulses or stimulation which come to the consciousness are never the same. Therefore, consciousness is always looking for no-change: quiet, serenity, peace of mind, eternity, security. Social security, insurance, old age pensions, medicine, and modern civilization developed through the character of consciousness. On the other hand, our subconscious maintains internal conditions such as temperature, blood sugar, amount of water, minerals, oxygen, and carbon dioxide and keeps them all constant. This is called *homeostasis*. In other words, one of the functions of subconsciousness is to maintain constancy. Therefore, the subconscious will have nothing to do if there is no change; it will be bored.

Here is a great paradox: consciousness wants no changes and subconsciousness wants changes. For example, I want a lasting job. I go to work every day at the same time, do the same job, and come home at the same time every day, every day. But soon I will become bored with the job. I'll want to change the job or my way of living. My consciousness tells me to keep the job, and my subconsciousness doesn't want it. When conscious and subconscious disagree with each other I cannot be happy. What shall I do?

This same paradox causes a great deal of trouble in marriage. At the beginning of a marriage, consciousness receives all new stimulation and the subconsciousness is challenged, so there is happiness. But life soon becomes monotonous. There is no challenge and the subconscious is not happy and begins to look for some changes. This is a danger sign. The wife and husband look at each other without excitement; life is boring. They look around for some excitement. Another mate comes into the picture which may bring the excitement that the subconscious wants.

How can we solve this great paradox in ourselves? We must create and find difference in sameness. We have to be creative. We have to continually improve our living and constantly explore our life to discover the deeper meaning of everything we encounter. For example, a wife should create new cooking techniques or recipes. If she cooks the same meals for 365 days, her husband will not be happy. A husband should plan their life to be bigger and deeper materially and spiritually.

Without this challenge of improvement and of being creative, the subconscious will soon be bored. When the subconscious mind is bored, life is dead; we become living corpses.

Have a dream in life and plan for it and work on it with constant faith in Infinity.

Message to the Macrobiotic Congress

Congratulations to you all who gathered here to discuss the future development of macrobiotics in North America. I appreciate your efforts, especially the person who organized this Congress and the one who helped him. I will not be able to attend this year's Congress because of my personal engagements; therefore, I asked a friend to bring you this message.

I travelled around the U.S.A. this summer lecturing on macrobiotics in over 15 cities. Macrobiotics is growing in the United States. I realized one tendency which I think most important. That is to say, there is an increased number of macrobiotic teachers, and they teach macrobiotics as their profession. In a way this is a great development. However, in a way, this is a beginning of the degradation of quality in macrobiotics. When doctors made medicine as their profession, the medical art became degraded. When medicine is a profession, healing is no more an art but a business. At this stage of macrobiotics, teachers are not degraded; they are very sincere people because they are not making money but barely sustain living. However, there are chances for them to degrade themselves. When does this happen? When they think of themselves as teachers.

What is the condition of a teacher? What is the difference between teachers and students? Usually people consider a person as a teacher one who has knowledge, experience, and persuasive ability in his field. I see one more condition. A teacher is one who sees the shortcomings of others. Because he sees one or more shortcomings of others, he can make judgments on others who may have an illness or unhappiness which is the result of their shortcoming, bad habit, or bad way of living. Therefore, a good teacher is one who sees the shortcomings of others and can give good advice to overcome the consequences. The best teacher is one who can teach how to change another's shortcomings. George Ohsawa was such a teacher. In any case, a teacher is one who sees the short-comings in others.

Then what is a student? A student is one who sees the shortcomings in himself. A student who sees few short-comings in himself is a beginning student. A student who sees over 10 shortcomings in himself is a better student. A student who sees over 100 shortcomings in himself is an ex-cellent student. In my opinion, the person who becomes happy is always a student, not a teacher. My wife, Cornelia-san, is a good teacher; she sees her students' shortcomings quickly and clearly and teaches how to correct them. How-ever, sometimes she is not a good student. When I taught her how to drive, she was a bad student. She didn't admit she was driving incorrectly when I told her. So I warned her that she would have an accident. Two days before this year's summer camp, she had an accident. She wrecked her new car and she couldn't stand up and walk for two days.

Therefore, I am giving this message as a warning to all sincere students of macrobiotics who want to be teachers. Don't try to be a teacher unless you are a good or excellent student of macrobiotics. When you are an excellent student you are a good teacher already.

However, at the stage of supreme judgment there is neither student nor teacher. There is only man in nature. Student and teacher are man-made concepts. Therefore when you reach supreme judgment, the above advice is not necessary of course.

Thanksgiving 1979

I give thanks to the Creator, who gave the universe the order

I give thanks for the sun, a source of warmth and energy; the moon, the source of rest; the stars, the source of guidance

I give thanks to light, air, water, green plants, and animals, without whom I wouldn't be here

I give thanks to all people that lived, are living, and will live in the future; without them I wouldn't have my necessities

I give thanks to my ancestors and my parents who originated my life in this world and nursed me

I give thanks to my brothers and sisters and children, who gave more meaning to my life

I give thanks to my wife, partners, and friends who corrected my mistakes, who encouraged my weakness, who betrayed my trust, worked against my plan, and lied on their promises – because they made me wiser and stronger

I give thanks to my teachers, from ancient to
    present, from East to West, whose teaching
    and example of living guide me
    to find meaning of life, the way of life,
    and the joy of living

I give thanks to difficulties and sicknesses I had,
    through which I learned the greatness of life

I give thanks to everything, including myself.

Life is wonderful.

The Author

Herman Aihara was born in Arita, a small town in southern Japan, on September 28, 1920. This town is famous for its production of porcelains called *Imari-ware* or *Kakiemon-ware;* Imari is the name of the port from which Arita porcelains were shipped to Europe (Germany, Holland, France) 200 years ago. Even though the porcelains were produced at Arita they were called *Imari-ware* because foreign merchants and others bought them at Imari.

His birth family was too poor to support ten children, and so at the age of nine Herman was adopted into an uncle's home in Tokyo. His family name was changed to Aihara. He grew up without knowing his actual mother. He was told who she was when she died, and at that time he returned to his native community for the first time.

There were many changes in his new environment. Accustomed to many brothers and sisters, he was an only child in his adoptive home and so he grew up alone. Although born at the quiet countryside in the spirit of craftsmanship, he now lived in a busy metropolis – the center of industry. His 'stepfather' owned a factory that produced iron materials for the national railways and telephone companies, and Herman chose metallurgical engineering as a life work. He was accepted by the school of engineering at the reputable Waseda University.

At this time he attended a lecture by George Ohsawa. Immediately he became more interested in the philosophy of yin and yang than metallurgy. As World War II began in 1942 he graduated with a bachelor's degree from Waseda. Illness kept him from military service. When the war ended, he recovered and began to attend Ohsawa's classes from time to time.

During this time, while working at his father's factory, he experienced a short marriage that ended in tragedy. Seeking help, Herman stayed a month at George Ohsawa's school and deeply absorbed his spirit and philosophy. Ohsawa was teaching macrobiotics with a new slogan – World Government – and appealing for young people to go out to other countries. Herman decided to go to America and start a new life.

In 1952 he arrived in San Francisco. He went to New York to meet Mr. and Mrs. Kushi, students of Ohsawa, and worked with them to establish macrobiotics there. Herman was elected president of the Ohsawa Foundation of New York. He and his new wife, another Ohsawa student, also managed two gift shops in New York until their move to Chico, California in 1961.

Since then the Aiharas have lived in California. After a short time as president of the Ohsawa Foundation of Los Angeles, Herman moved to San Francisco where he founded and became president of the George Ohsawa Macrobiotic Foundation in 1970. In 1974 he moved the Foundation to Oroville, a small town in northern California. In this quiet atmosphere with its proximity to the macrobiotic community in the Chico area, Herman has been at home. His productivity as an author, translator, lecturer, spiritual and health advisor, and family man has thrived in this environment.

Late in the evening, after dinner at the Foundation, a small light can be seen burning on his desk from across the street. A quiet, serious, but humorous man with white hair is always working, always studying.

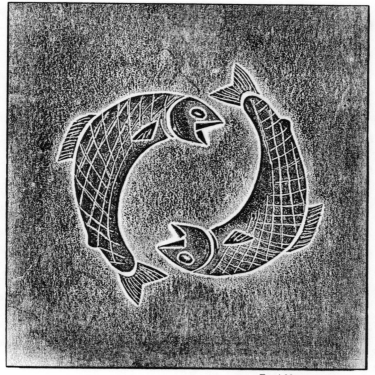

Fumi Matsumoto